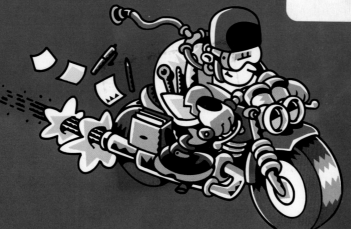

Anatomy

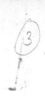

Series editor
Daniel Horton-Szar
BSc (Hons)
United Medical and Dental
Schools of Guy's and
St Thomas's Hospitals
(UMDS),
London

Faculty advisor
Ian Whitmore
MD, MB BS, LRCP, MRCS
Visiting Professor of
Anatomy,
Stanford University, USA,
Pretoria and
Johannesburg
Universities, South Africa

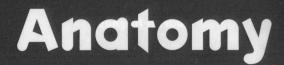

Anatomy

Phillip Ameerally
BDs
United Medical and
Dental Schools of Guy's
and St Thomas's
Hospitals (UMDS),
London

Nik Suhaila
Year 1996/2001
bought on : 20/4/00

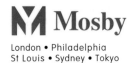 Mosby

London • Philadelphia
St Louis • Sydney • Tokyo

Publisher	**Dianne Zack**
Managing Editor	**Louise Crowe**
Development Editors	**Filipa Maia**
	Marion Jowett
Project Manager	**Linda Horrell**
Designer	**Greg Smith**
Layout	**Marie McNestry**
Illustration Management	**Danny Pyne**
Illustrators	**Jenni Miller**
	Lynda Payne
	Danny Pyne
	Mike Saiz
	Marion Tasker
	Annette Whalley
Cover Design	**Greg Smith**
Production	**Gudrun Hughes**
Index	**Janine Ross**

ISBN 0 7234 2995 2

Copyright © Mosby International Ltd, 1998.

Published by Mosby, an imprint of Mosby International Ltd, Lynton House, 7–12 Tavistock Square, London WC1H 9LB, UK.

Printed in Barcelona, Spain, by Grafos S.A. Arte sobre papel, 1998.
Text set in Crash Course—VAG Light; captions in Crash Course—VAG Thin.

Cataloguing in Publication Data
Catalogue records for this book are available from the British Library and the US Library of Congress.

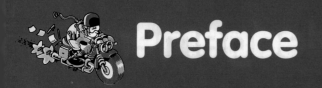

Preface

Anatomy is a wonderful and exciting subject but it is often very intimidating to medical students. Not only do students have to learn an entirely new vocabulary, but they also have to cover a large volume of work in a short space of time. This book has been written with this in mind.

We have presented anatomy in a simple, clear, and concise manner with the aid of numerous diagrams, tables, and bulleted lists. Information should be easy to obtain without the need to read through large volumes of text. Clinical information has also been included to demonstrate the importance of anatomy in clinical medicine and to further stimulate students' interest. Comprehension check boxes and hints and tips boxes are present throughout to aid memory.

The final section of the book contains 40 multiple choice questions and answers, 12 short answer questions with model answers, and 10 essay questions which will help final revision.

Phillip Ameerally

OK, no-one ever said medicine was going to be easy, but the thing is, there are very few parts of this enormous subject that are actually difficult to understand. The problem for most of us is the sheer volume of information that must be absorbed before each round of exams. It's not fun when time is getting short and you realize that: a) you really should have done a bit more work by now; and b) there are large gaps in your lecture notes that you meant to copy up but never quite got round to.

This series has been designed and written by senior medical students and doctors with recent experience of basic medical science exams. We've brought together all the information you need into compact, manageable volumes that integrate basic science with clinical skills. There is a consistent structure and layout across the series, and every title is checked for accuracy by senior faculty members from medical schools across the UK.

I hope this book makes things a little easier!

Danny Horton-Szar
Series Editor (Basic Medical Sciences)

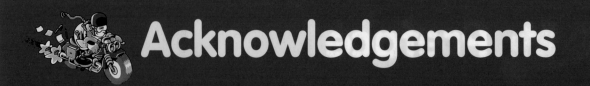

Acknowledgements

Figure Credits
Figure 5.29 (upper part from *Clinical Examination 3e*, by Dr O Epstein, Dr D Perkin, Dr D de Bono, and Dr J Cookson, Mosby International, 1997; lower part from *Integrated Pharmacology* by Professor C Page, Dr M Curtris, Dr M Sutter, Dr M Walker, and Dr B Hoffman, Mosby International, 1997).

Contents

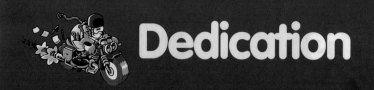

Dedication

To Macadeen and Shirley Ameerally
who both worked very hard to get me where I am today,
and to Debra, Tony, Andrew, and the new generation

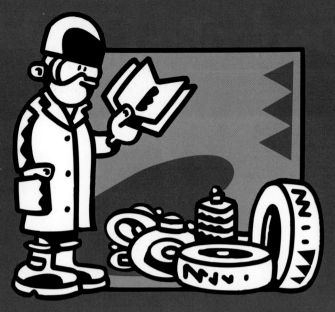

ANATOMY

ANATOMY

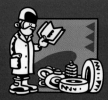

1. Basic Concepts of Anatomy

DESCRIPTIVE ANATOMICAL TERMS

The anatomical position

This is a standard position used in anatomy and clinical medicine to allow accurate and consistent description of one body part in relation to another (Fig. 1.1):

- The body is upright, legs together, and directed forwards.
- The palms are turned forward, with the thumbs laterally.

Regions of the body

Note: the upper limb is composed of the scapular region, the arm, the forearm, and the hand; the lower limb is composed of the gluteal region, the thigh, the leg, and the foot.

Fig. 1.1 Anatomical position and regions of the body.

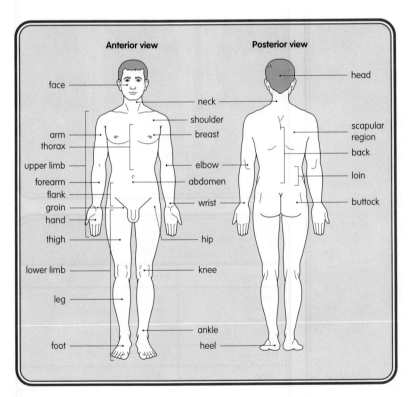

Anterior view   Posterior view

face
neck
shoulder
arm
breast
thorax
upper limb
elbow
forearm
abdomen
flank
groin
hand
wrist
thigh
hip
lower limb
knee
leg
ankle
foot
heel

head
scapular region
back
loin
buttock

Anatomical planes

These comprise the following (Fig. 1.2):

- The median sagittal plane is the vertical plane passing through the midline of the body from the front to the back. Any plane parallel to this is termed paramedian or sagittal.
- Coronal planes are vertical planes perpendicular to the sagittal planes.
- Horizontal or transverse planes lie at right angles to both the sagittal and coronal planes.

Terms of position

The terms of position commonly used in clinical practice and anatomy are illustrated in Fig. 1.3.

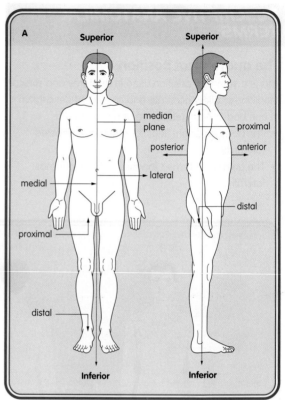

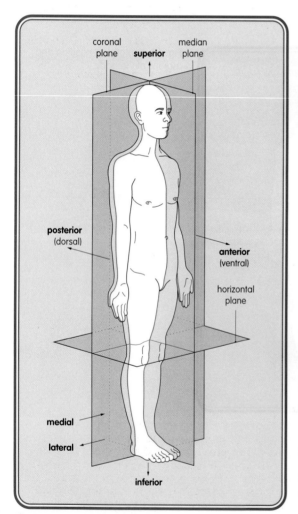

Fig. 1.2 Anatomical planes.

B	Classification of terms commonly used in anatomy and clinical practice	
Position		**Description**
anterior		in front of another structure
posterior		behind another structure
superior		above another structure
inferior		below another structure
superficial		closer to the body surface
deep		further away from the body surface
medial		closer to the median plane
lateral		further away from the median plane
proximal		closer to the trunk or origin
distal		further away from the trunk or origin

Fig. 1.3 Relationship and comparison (A) and classification (B) of terms of position commonly used in anatomy and clinical practice.

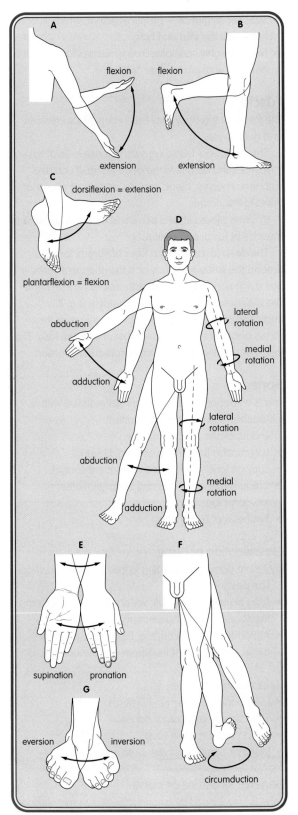

Terms of movement

Various terms are used to describe movements of the body (Fig. 1.4):

- Flexion—movement in a sagittal plane which reduces the angle at the joint (except at the ankle joint), e.g. bending the elbow.
- Extension—increases the angle at joints in the same plane.
- Abduction—movement away from the median plane.
- Adduction—movement towards the median plane.
- Supination—movement, e.g. lateral rotation of the forearm, causing the palm to face anteriorly.
- Pronation—movement, e.g. medial rotation of the forearm, causing the palm to face posteriorly.
- Eversion—turning the sole of the foot outwards.
- Inversion—turning the sole of the foot inwards.
- Rotation—movement of part of the body around its long axis.
- Circumduction—combination movement.

Fig. 1.4 Terms of movement.
(A) Flexion and extension of forearm at elbow joint.
(B) Flexion and extension of leg at knee joint.
(C) Dorsiflexion and plantarflexion of foot at ankle joint.
(D) Abduction and adduction of right limbs and rotation of left limbs at shoulder and hip joints, respectively.
(E) Pronation and supination of forearm at radioulnar joints.
(F) Circumduction (circular movement) of lower limb at hip joint.
(G) Inversion and eversion of foot at subtalar and transverse tarsal joints.

BASIC STRUCTURES OF ANATOMY

Skin

The skin completely covers the body surface and is the largest organ of the body. The functions of the skin include:

- Protection from ultraviolet light and mechanical, chemical, and thermal insults.
- Sensations including pain, temperature, touch, and pressure.
- Thermoregulation.
- Metabolic functions, e.g. vitamin D synthesis.

The skin is composed of the following (Fig. 1.5):

- The epidermis. This forms a protective waterproof barrier. It consists of epithelium, which is continuously being shed and replaced, and is avascular.
- The dermis. This supports the epidermis and has a rich network of vessels and nerves. It is composed mainly of collagen fibres with elastic fibres, giving the skin its elasticity.
- The hypodermis or superficial fascia. This acts as a shock-absorbing layer below the skin.

The skin appendages include:

- Hairs—highly modified, keratinized structures.
- Sweat glands—produce sweat, which plays a role in thermoregulation.

- Sebaceous glands—produce sebum, which lubricates the skin and hair.
- Nails—highly specialized appendages found on the dorsal end of each finger and toe.

Fascia

The fascia of the body may be divided into superficial and deep layers.

The superficial fascia consists of loose areolar tissue that unites the dermis to the deep fascia. It contains cutaneous nerves, blood vessels, and lymphatics that travel to the dermis.

In some places sheets of muscle lie in the fascia, e.g. muscles of facial expression.

The deep fascia forms a layer of fibrous tissue around the limbs and body and the deep structures. It has a rich nerve supply and is therefore very sensitive. The thickness of the fascia varies widely: e.g. it is thickened in the iliotibial tract but very thin over the rectus abdominis muscle and absent over the face. The fascia determines the pattern of spread of infection.

Bone

This is a specialized form of connective tissue with a mineralized extracellular component.

The functions of bone include:

- Locomotion (by serving as a rigid lever).
- Support (giving soft tissue permanent shape).
- Calcium homoeostasis and storage of other inorganic ions.
- Synthesis of blood cells.

Classification of bone

Bones are classified according to their position and shape.

The position can be:

- Axial skeleton, e.g. skull, vertebral column including the sacrum, ribs, and sternum.
- Appendicular skeleton, e.g. hip bones, pectoral girdle, and bones of the upper and lower limbs.

Types of shape include:

- Long bones, e.g. femur, humerus.
- Short bones, e.g. carpal bones.
- Flat bones, e.g. skull vault.
- Irregular bones, e.g. vertebrae.

General structure of bone

Bone is surrounded by a connective-tissue membrane called the periosteum (Fig. 1.6). This is continuous with

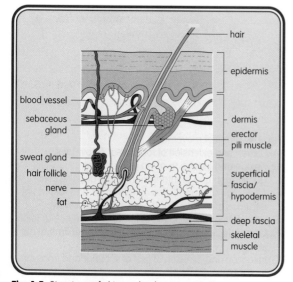

Fig. 1.5 Structure of skin and subcutaneous tissue.

muscle attachments, joint capsules, and the deep fascia. There is an outer fibrous layer and an inner cellular layer. The inner layer is vascular and provides the underlying bone with nutrition. It also contains progenitor cells, which may differentiate into osteoblasts when required.

After a fracture, the cells of the periosteum differentiate into osteoblasts and form a cuff of bone around the fracture site. This helps to stabilize the bone while it heals from the inside.

Bone includes the following components:
- The outer compact layer or cortical bone provides great strength and rigidity.
- The cancellous or spongy bone consists of a network of trabeculae arranged to resist external forces.
- The medullary cavity of long bones and the interstices of cancellous bone are filled with red (haematopoietic) or yellow (fatty) marrow. At birth virtually all the bone marrow is red, but this is replaced by yellow marrow—only the ribs, sternum, vertebrae, clavicle, pelvis, and skull bones contain red marrow in adult life.
- The endosteum is a single-cellular osteogenic layer lining the inner surface of bone.

Blood supply of bones

There are two main sources of blood supply to bone:
- A major nutrient artery that supplies the marrow.
- Vessels from the periosteum.

The periosteal supply to bone assumes greater importance in the elderly. Extensive stripping of the periosteum, e.g. during surgery or following trauma, may result in bone death.

Joints

These are unions between bones (Fig. 1.7).

Synovial joints

These have the following features:
- The bone ends are covered by hyaline articular cartilage.
- The joint is surrounded by a fibrous capsule.
- A synovial membrane lines the inner aspect of the joint, except where there is cartilage, and contains synovial fluid, which lubricates the joint and transports nutrients, especially to the cartilage.
- Some synovial joints, e.g. the temporomandibular joints, are divided into two cavities by an articular disc.

Blood supply of joints

A vascular plexus around the epiphysis provides the joint with a very good blood supply.

Nerve supply of joints

According to Hilton's law, the motor nerve to a muscle tends to give a branch to the joint that the muscle moves and another branch to the skin over the joint. The capsule and ligaments are supplied by afferent nerve endings including pain fibres. The synovial membrane contains few pain fibres and there are no afferent fibres in articular cartilage; joint pain is therefore poorly localized.

Stability of joints

Stability is achieved by the following components:
- Bony—e.g. in a firm ball-and-socket joint such as the hip joint, bony contours contribute to stability.

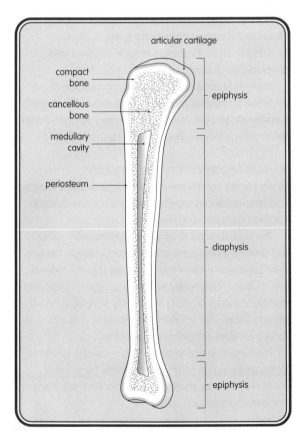

Fig. 1.6 Long bone and its components.

- Ligaments—these are important in most joints and act mainly to prevent excessive movement.
- Muscles—these are an important stabilizing factor in most joints.

Muscles and tendons

Skeletal muscles are aggregations of contractile fibres that move large structures such as the skeleton.

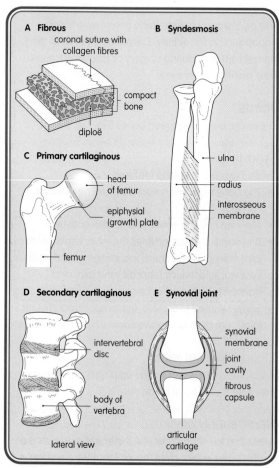

Fig. 1.7 Types of joints.
(A) Fibrous (bones are united by fibrous tissue, as in sutures of the skull).
(B) Syndesmosis (bones are joined by a sheet of fibrous tissue).
(C) Primary cartilaginous (where bone and hyaline cartilage meet).
(D) Secondary cartilaginous (articular surfaces are covered by a thin lamina of hyaline cartilage; the hyaline laminae are united by fibrocartilage).
(E) Synovial joint.

Muscles are attached to bone by tendons at their origin and insertion.

Muscle action

Muscles can be classified according to their action:
- Prime mover—the muscle is the major muscle responsible for a particular movement, e.g. brachialis is the prime mover in flexing the arm.
- Antagonist—any muscle that opposes the action of the prime mover: it relaxes, but in a controlled manner, to assist the prime mover , e.g. triceps in flexion of the elbow.
- Fixator—prime mover and antagonist acting together to 'fix' a joint, e.g. muscles holding the scapula steady when deltoid moves the humerus.
- Synergist—prevents unwanted movement in an intermediate joint, e.g extensors of the carpus contract to fix the wrist joint, allowing the long flexors of the fingers to function effectively.

Muscle design

Muscle fibres may be either parallel or oblique to the line of pull of the whole muscle.

Parallel fibres allow maximal range of mobility. These muscles may be quadrangular, fusiform, bicipital, or strap. Examples include sartorius and sternocleidomastoid.

Oblique fibres increase the force generated at the expense of reduced mobility. These muscles may be unipennate, bipennate, or multipennate. Examples include flexor pollicis longus, dorsal interossei, and deltoid.

Muscle organization and function

Motor nerves control the contraction of skeletal muscle. Each motor neuron together with the muscle fibres it supplies constitutes a motor unit.

The size of motor units varies considerably: where fine precise movements are required, a single neuron may supply only a few muscle fibres, e.g. the extrinsic eye muscles; conversely, in the large gluteus maximus muscle, a single neuron may supply several hundred muscle fibres. The smaller the size of the motor unit, the more precise the movements possible.

The force generated by a skeletal muscle is related to the cross-sectional area of its fibres. For a fixed volume of muscle, shorter fibres produce more force but less shortening.

Muscle attachments

The ends of muscles are attached to bone, cartilage, and ligaments by tendons. Some flat muscles are attached by a flattened tendon, an aponeurosis.

When symmetrical muscle fibres unite at an angle, e.g. in mylohyoid muscle, a raphe is formed.

When tendons cross joints, they are often enclosed in a synovial sheath, a layer of connective tissue lined by a synovial membrane and lubricated by synovial fluid.

Bursae are sacs of connective tissue filled with synovial fluid which lie between tendons and bony areas, acting as cushioning devices.

Nerves

The nervous system is divided into the central nervous system and the peripheral nervous system: the central nervous system is composed of the brain and spinal cord; the peripheral nervous system consists of the cranial and spinal nerves, and their distribution. The nervous system may also be divided into the somatic and autonomic nervous systems.

The conducting cells of the nervous system are termed neurons. A typical motor neuron consists of a cell body which contains the nucleus and gives off a single axon and numerous dendrites (Fig. 1.8). The cell bodies of most neurons are located within the central nervous system, where they aggregate to form nuclei. Cell bodies in the peripheral nervous system aggregate in ganglia.

Axons are the nerve fibres and conduct action potentials generated in the cell body, to influence other neurons or affect organs. They may be myelinated or non-myelinated.

Most nerves in the peripheral nervous system are bundles of motor, sensory, and autonomic axons. The region of the head is largely supplied by the 12 cranial nerves. The remainder of the trunk and the limbs are segmentally supplied by the spinal nerves.

The importance of the myelin sheath is well illustrated in multiple sclerosis, where focal loss of myelin leads to severe disability.

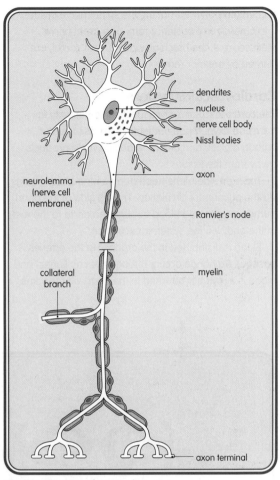

Fig. 1.8 Structure of a typical neuron.

Spinal nerves

There are 31 pairs of spinal nerves: eight cervical, 12 thoracic, five lumbar, five sacral, and the coccygeal nerve. The spinal cord ends at the lower border of the first lumbar vertebra in the adult. Below this, the nerve roots of the cord form a vertical bundle, the cauda equina.

Each spinal nerve is formed by the union of the anterior and posterior roots (Fig. 1.9):

- The anterior root contains motor fibres for skeletal muscles. Those from T1 to L2 contain sympathetic fibres; S2 to S4 also contain parasympathetic fibres.
- The posterior root contains sensory fibres whose cell bodies are in the posterior root ganglion.

Immediately after formation, the spinal nerve divides into anterior and posterior rami. The great nerve plexuses, e.g. the brachial, lumbar, and sacral, are formed by anterior rami.

Cardiovascular system

The cardiovascular system functions principally to transport oxygen and nutrients to the tissues and carbon dioxide and other metabolic waste products away from the tissues.

The right side of the heart pumps blood to the lungs via the pulmonary circulation. The left side of the heart pumps oxygenated blood through the aorta to the rest of the body via the systemic circulation.

Blood is distributed to the organs via the arteries, gaseous exchange occurs through the capillaries, and blood is eventually returned to the heart via the veins.

Valves in the low-pressure venous system are required to prevent back-flow of blood. Loss of competence of the lower-limb valves results in varicose veins.

Anastomosis

This is a communication between two vessels. Normally little flow of blood occurs through anastomoses; however, if an artery is occluded, the anastomoses assume greater importance in helping to maintain the circulation to an organ. If an artery is slowly occluded, new vessels develop (collaterals), forming an alternative pathway.

When such communications are absent between arteries, the vessel is known as an end artery. Occlusion in these vessels leads to necrosis, e.g. in the central artery of the retina.

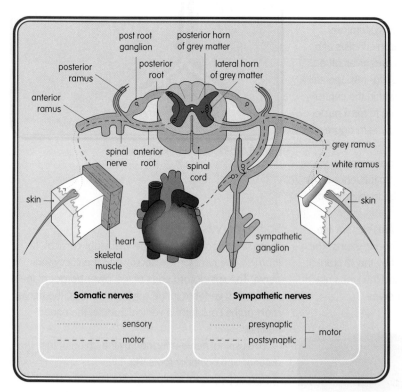

Fig. 1.9 Components of a typical spinal nerve.

Lymphatics

Fig. 1.10 illustrates the lymphatic system in man.

Fluid moves into the tissues at the arterial end of the circulation and most is returned at the venous end. Excess fluid is drained into the lymphatic system as lymph, which is ultimately returned to the venous system and the right side of the heart.

Lymph also transports foreign materials to lymph nodes, initiating an immune response, and absorption of fats in the gastrointestinal tract is into the lymphatic system.

Lymphatics are found in all tissues except the central nervous system, eyeball, internal ear, cartilage, bone, and epidermis of the skin.

Fig. 1.10 The lymphatic system.

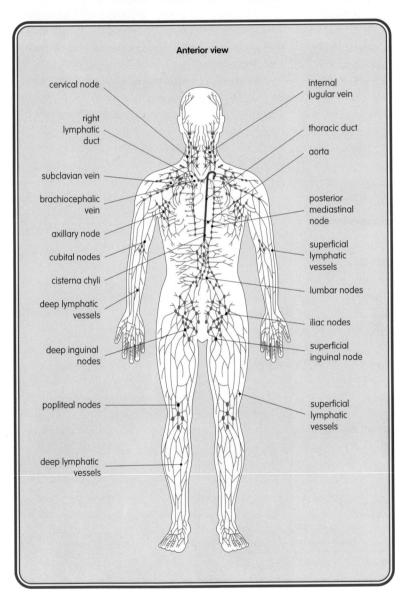

Anterior view

cervical node

right lymphatic duct

subclavian vein

brachiocephalic vein

axillary node

cubital nodes

cisterna chyli

deep lymphatic vessels

deep inguinal nodes

popliteal nodes

deep lymphatic vessels

internal jugular vein

thoracic duct

aorta

posterior mediastinal node

superficial lymphatic vessels

lumbar nodes

iliac nodes

superficial inguinal node

superficial lymphatic vessels

- List the anatomical terms.
- What are the anatomical planes?
- Describe the terms of position and movement.
- Discuss the structure of bone.
- Describe the structure of muscle and nerves.
- Outline the layout of the cardiovascular and lymphatic systems.

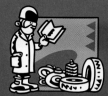

2. The Upper Limb

REGIONS AND COMPONENTS OF THE UPPER LIMB

The upper limb is joined to the trunk by the shoulder or pectoral girdle. The shoulder region is the area around the shoulder joint and girdle. The arm lies between the shoulder and the elbow. The forearm lies between the elbow and the wrist. The hands join the forearm at the wrist.

The shoulder girdle is composed of the scapula and clavicle, which articulate at the acromioclavicular joint. The sternoclavicular joint is the only joint between the shoulder girdle and the axial skeleton, and connects the shoulder girdle to the axial skeleton. All the remaining attachments to the axial skeleton are muscular. The humerus lies in the arm and articulates with the scapula and with the ulna and radius. The radius articulates with the hand at the wrist joint.

The subclavian artery is the major arterial supply of the upper limb. It arises from the brachiocephalic trunk on the right side and directly from the aorta on the left side. It continues as the axillary artery and then as the brachial artery, which divides into the radial and ulnar arteries to supply the forearm and hand.

Blood is returned to the axillary vein, which becomes the subclavian vein. Superficial veins drain into the axillary vein.

The nerve supply to the upper limb is derived from the brachial plexus: the anterior compartments are supplied by the median, musculocutaneous, and ulnar nerves; the posterior compartments are supplied by the radial nerve.

SURFACE ANATOMY AND SUPERFICIAL STRUCTURES

Surface anatomy
Surface anatomy of the shoulder region is shown in Fig. 2.1.

Scapula
The tip of the coracoid process can be felt on deep palpation in the lateral part of the deltopectoral triangle—a small depression situated below the outer third of the clavicle, bounded by the pectoralis major and deltoid muscles. The deltoid muscle forms the smooth round curve of the shoulder.

The acromion process is easily located in its subcutaneous position.

The crest of the scapula may be palpated and followed to its medial border. The inferior angle of the scapula can be palpated opposite the T7 vertebral spine.

Axilla and axillary folds
The anterior and posterior axillary folds may be palpated. The head of the humerus can be palpated through the floor of the axilla.

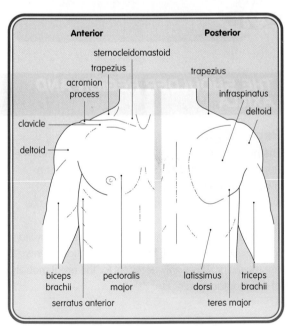

Fig. 2.1 Surface anatomy of the anterior and posterior views of the shoulder region.

Elbow region

The medial and lateral epicondyles of the humerus and the olecranon process of the ulna can be palpated. The head of the radius can be palpated in a depression on the posterior aspect of the extended elbow, distal to the lateral epicondyle. The cubital fossa lies anterior to the elbow joint. The biceps brachii tendon is palpable as it enters the fossa.

The brachial artery may be palpated as it passes down the medial aspect of the arm.

The styloid processes of the radius and ulna may be palpated at the wrist.

Superficial venous drainage

The dorsal and the palmar veins drain into the dorsal venous network (Fig. 2.2). From this the medial basilic

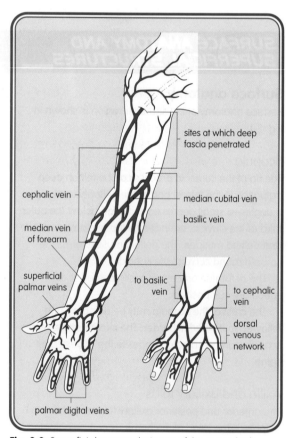

Fig. 2.2 Superficial venous drainage of the upper limb.

Labels on figure:
- sites at which deep fascia penetrated
- cephalic vein
- median cubital vein
- basilic vein
- median vein of forearm
- superficial palmar veins
- to basilic vein
- to cephalic vein
- dorsal venous network
- palmar digital veins

and lateral cephalic veins arise and ascend in the forearm to the arm. The basilic vein passes to halfway up the arm, pierces the deep fascia, and drains into the brachial vein. The cephalic vein passes onto the anterolateral aspect of the forearm and communicates with the basilic vein in the median cubital vein—this last vein is usually easy to identify and is frequently used for venepuncture. The cephalic vein continues up the arm laterally to the deltopectoral groove and then to the infraclavicular fossa, where it drains into the axillary vein.

Lymphatic drainage

Lymphatics in the hand coalesce to form trunks that ascend the forearm and the arm with the cephalic and basilic veins and the deep veins. Vessels accompanying the cephalic vein drain into the infraclavicular nodes or the axillary nodes. Some vessels along the basilic vein are interrupted at the elbow by a supratrochlear node, but ultimately all drain into the axillary nodes. Superficial vessels from the shoulder region drain into the axillary nodes.

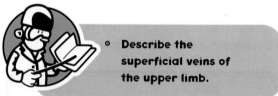

○ **Describe the superficial veins of the upper limb.**

THE SHOULDER REGION AND AXILLA

Pectoral girdle

The pectoral girdle (clavicle and scapula) suspends the upper limb whilst the clavicle holds the upper limb away from the trunk (Fig. 2.3). The girdle itself is suspended from the head and neck by the trapezius muscle.

It articulates directly with the axial skeleton only via the sternoclavicular joint; the remaining attachments are muscular. This partly accounts for the great mobility of the shoulder girdle.

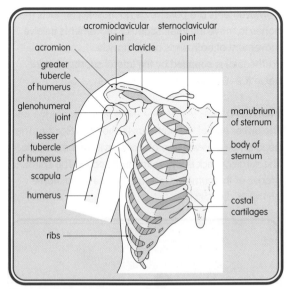

Fig. 2.3 Skeleton of the pectoral girdle.

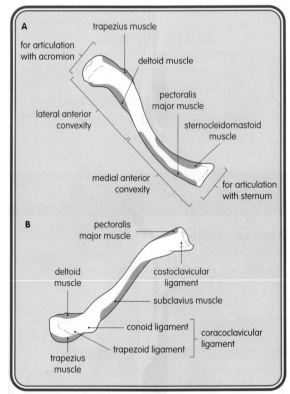

Fig. 2.4 Superior (A) and inferior (B) aspects of the right clavicle and its muscular attachments.

Clavicle

The clavicle is subcutaneous and articulates with the sternum medially and with the acromion process of the scapula laterally (Fig. 2.4). Fracture of the clavicle is common and usually occurs at the junction of the outer and middle thirds.

Scapula

The scapula is a triangular flat bone lying on the posterior thoracic wall. It has superior, medial and lateral borders, and superior and inferior angles (Fig. 2.5). The glenoid cavity articulates with the head of the humerus. The coracoid process projects upwards and forwards above the glenoid cavity and provides attachment for muscles and ligaments.

The subscapular fossa lies on the anterior surface; the supraspinous and infraspinous fossae are on the posterior surface, divided by the spine of the scapula, which expands laterally as the acromion.

Joints of the pectoral girdle
Sternoclavicular joint

This is an atypical synovial joint because the articular surfaces are covered by fibrocartilage, not hyaline cartilage. A capsule surrounds the joint and is reinforced by anterior and posterior sternoclavicular ligaments. The costoclavicular ligament also stabilizes the joint. An articular disc is attached to the capsule, dividing the joint into two cavities.

As the lateral end of the clavicle moves, its medial end moves in the opposite direction, moving around the costoclavicular ligament.

The joint is supplied by the medial supraclavicular nerve (C3–C4) from the cervical plexus.

Acromioclavicular joint

This is where the lateral end of the clavicle articulates with the medial border of the acromion. It is an atypical synovial joint, the articular surfaces being fibrocartilage. A weak capsule surrounds the articular surfaces. It is reinforced by the acromioclavicular ligament superiorly. The coracoclavicular ligament is very strong and is the major factor in joint stability.

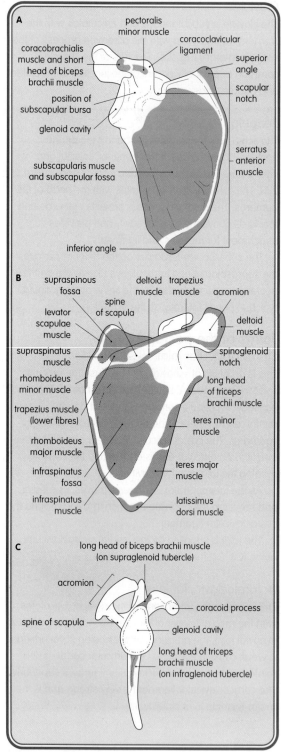

Fig. 2.5 Ventral (A), dorsal (B), and lateral (C) aspects of the right scapula and its muscular attachments.

Movements are passive as no muscle connects the bones to move the joint. Scapular movements involve movement at both ends of the clavicle.

The joint is supplied by the lateral supraclavicular nerve (C3–C4).

Humerus

The upper end of the humerus is shown in Fig. 2.6. The head articulates with the glenoid cavity of the scapula. The surgical neck is where fractures occur. The spiral groove of the humerus is related to the radial nerve.

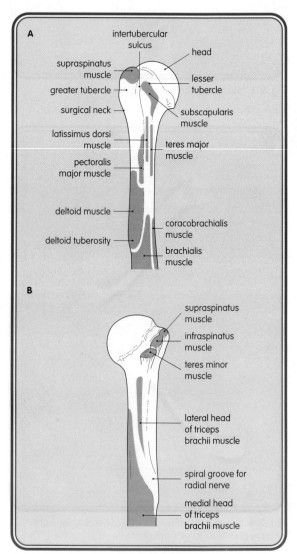

Fig. 2.6 (A) Anterior and (B) posterior views of the upper end of the humerus and its muscle attachments.

Muscles of the upper limb

Fig. 2.7 outlines the major muscles of the upper limb.

Major muscles of the upper limb			
Name of muscle (nerve supply)	Origin	Insertion	Action
latissimus dorsi (thoracordorsal nerve)	iliac crest, lumbar fascia, spinal processes of lower six thoracic vertebrae, lower ribs, scapula	floor of bicipital groove of humerus	extends, adducts, and medially rotates arm
levator scapulae (C3 and C4 and dorsal scapular nerve)	transverse processes of C1–C4	medial border of scapula	elevates medial part of scapula
rhomboideus minor (dorsal scapular nerve)	ligamentum nuchae, spines of C7 and T1	medial border of scapula	elevates medial border of scapula
rhomboideus major (dorsal scapular nerve)	spines of T2–T5	medial border of scapula	elevates medial border of scapula
trapezius (spinal part of XI nerve and C3 and C4)	occipital bone, ligamentum nuchae, thoracic vertebrae, spinal processes	lateral third of clavicle, acromion, spine of scapula	elevates scapula, pulls scapula medially and pulls medial border of scapula downward
subclavius (nerve to subclavius)	first costal cartilage	clavicle	depresses clavicle
pectoralis major (medial and lateral pectoral nerves)	clavicle, sternum, upper six costal cartilages	lateral lip of bicipital groove of humerus	adducts arm and rotates it medially
pectoralis minor (medial pectoral nerve)	third, fourth, and fifth ribs	coracoid process of scapula	depresses point of shoulder protracts shoulder
serratus anterior (long thoracic nerve)	upper eight ribs	medial border and inferior angle of scapula	pulls scapula forwards and rotates it
deltoid (axillary nerve)	clavicle, acromion, spine of scapula	lateral surface of humerus	abducts, flexes and medially rotates, extends, and laterally rotates arm
supraspinatus (suprascapular nerve)	supraspinous fossa of scapula	greater tuberosity of humerus, capsule of shoulder joint	abducts arm
subscapularis (upper and lower subscapular nerves)	subscapular fossa	lesser tuberosity of humerus	medially rotates arm
teres major (lower subscapular nerve)	lateral border of scapula	bicipital groove of humerus	medially rotates and adducts arm
teres minor (axillary nerve)	lateral border of scapula	greater tuberosity of humerus, capsule of shoulder joint	laterally rotates arm
infraspinatus (suprascapular nerve)	infraspinous fossa of scapula	greater tuberosity of humerus, capsule of shoulder joint	laterally rotates arm

Fig. 2.7 Major muscles of the upper limb.

Rotator cuff

The rotator cuff consists of the subscapularis, supraspinatus, infraspinatus, and teres minor. The tendons of these muscles surround the shoulder joint on all sides except inferiorly and blend with the capsule. They help to keep the large humeral head applied to the shallow glenoid cavity.

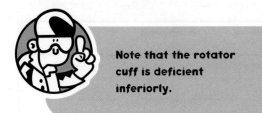

Note that the rotator cuff is deficient inferiorly.

Clavipectoral fascia

This is a strong sheet of connective tissue that encloses the subclavius and is attached to the clavicle. Below, it splits to enclose pectoralis minor and continues as the suspensory ligament of the axilla.

The following structures pass through the clavipectoral fascia:

- Cephalic vein.
- Thoracoacromial artery.
- Lymphatic vessels from the infraclavicular node.
- Lateral pectoral nerve.

Quadrangular and triangular spaces

A number of spaces are formed by the muscles and bones in the axillary region (Fig. 2.8)

Shoulder joint

Here there is articulation between the glenoid cavity of the scapula and the head of the humerus (Fig. 2.9). It is a multiaxial ball-and-socket synovial joint. A rim of fibrocartilage is attached to the margins of the glenoid cavity, the glenoid labrum.

The capsule surrounds the joint and is attached to the margins of the glenoid labrum and to the humerus around the anatomical neck. A gap in the anterior part of the capsule allows communication between the synovial cavity and subscapular bursa. The capsule is strong but loose, allowing great mobility. It is strengthened by the tendons of the rotator cuff. The long tendon of biceps brachii lies intracapsular and extrasynovial. The synovial membrane lines the capsule and part of the neck of the humerus. It communicates with the subscapular bursa and invests the long head of biceps brachii in a tubular sleeve.

The glenohumeral ligaments are three thickenings that slightly strengthen the capsule. The capsule is also reinforced by the strong coracohumeral ligament. The coracoacromial ligament forms an arch above the joint and prevents superior dislocation.

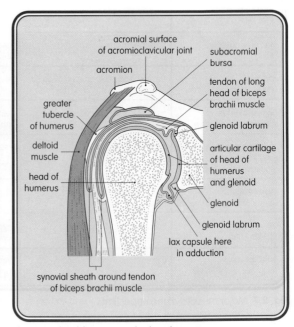

Fig. 2.8 Quadrangular and triangular spaces.

Fig. 2.9 Shoulder joint and related structures.

The shoulder joint is inherently unstable owing to the very large head of the humerus compared with the shallow glenoid cavity. Factors stabilizing the shoulder joint are the glenoid labrum, all the ligaments and the muscles supporting the joint.

The movements at the shoulder joint and the muscles performing them are described in Fig. 2.10. The movement of abduction deserves special mention: a maximum of 120 degrees of abduction is possible at the glenohumeral joint. Further movement is obtained by rotating the inferior angle of the scapula laterally and anteriorly, turning the glenoid cavity upwards. This is achieved by serratus anterior and trapezius.

Axilla

The major vessels of the upper limb leave the neck to enter the apex of the axilla.

The contents of the axilla are shown in Fig. 2.11 and include:

- Axillary artery.
- Axillary vein.
- Brachial plexus.
- Axillary lymph nodes.

Axillary artery

This is a continuation of the third part of the subclavian artery and commences at the outer border of the first rib. It is invested in fascia, with the brachial plexus,

Movements of the shoulder joint and the muscles performing them	
Movement	**Muscles**
flexion	pectoralis major, anterior fibres of deltoid
extension	posterior fibres of deltoid, latissimus dorsi, teres major
abduction	deltoid, supraspinatus
adduction	pectoralis major, latissimus dorsi, subscapularis, teres major, infraspinatus
lateral rotation	infraspinatus, teres minor, posterior fibres of deltoid
medial rotation	pectoralis major, anterior fibres of deltoid, latissimus dorsi, teres major, subscapularis
circumduction	varying combinations of flexion, extension, abduction, and adduction muscles

Fig. 2.10 Movements of the shoulder joint and the muscles performing them.

Fig. 2.11 Contents and muscular boundaries of the axilla.

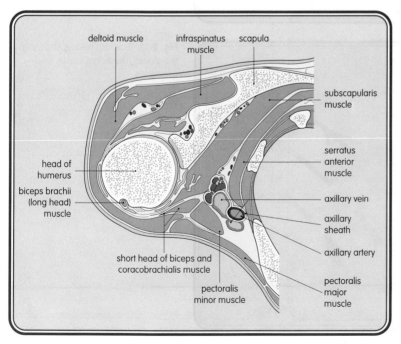

derived from the prevertebral fascia. The axillary artery becomes the brachial artery at the lower border of teres major. It is divided into three parts by pectoralis minor (Fig. 2.12):

- The first part has one branch—the superior thoracic artery.
- The second part has two branches—the thoracoacromial and the lateral thoracic arteries.
- The third part has three branches—the subscapular and the anterior and posterior circumflex humeral arteries.

Axillary vein

This is a continuation of the venae comitantes of the brachial artery, which are joined by the basilic vein. It commences at the lower border of teres major and ascends through the axilla medial to the axillary artery. At the outer border of the first rib it becomes the subclavian vein.

Brachial plexus

This is formed from five roots, these being the anterior rami of C5–C8 and T1 spinal nerves (Figs 2.13 and 2.14).

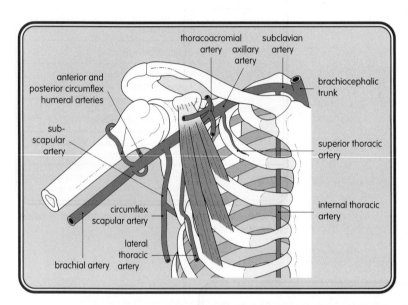

Fig. 2.12 Axillary artery and its branches.

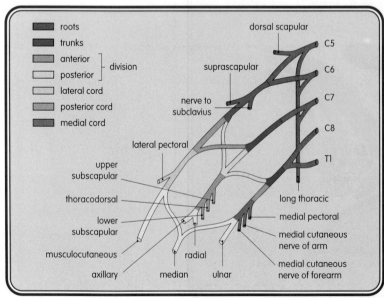

Fig. 2.13 Brachial plexus showing the trunks, divisions, cords, and branches.

Branches of the brachial plexus and their distribution	
Branches	**Distribution**
Roots	
dorsal scapular nerve (C5)	rhomboid minor, rhomboid major, levator scapulae muscles
long thoracic nerve (C5–C7)	serratus anterior muscle
Upper trunk	
suprascapular nerve (C5, C6)	supraspinatus and infraspinatus muscles
nerve to subclavius	subclavius muscle
Lateral cord	
lateral pectoral nerve (C5–C7)	pectoralis major muscle
musculocutaneous nerve (C5–C7)	coracobrachialis, biceps brachii, brachialis muscles, and skin along lateral border of forearm (lateral cutaneous nerve of forearm)
lateral root of median nerve	
Posterior cord	
upper subscapular nerve (C5–C6)	subscapularis muscle
thoracodorsal nerve (C6–C8)	latissimus dorsi muscle
lower subscapular nerve (C5–C6)	subscapularis and teres major muscles
axillary nerve (C5–C6)	deltoid and teres minor muscles; skin over lower half of deltoid muscle (upper lateral cutaneous nerve of arm)
radial nerve (C5–C8, T1)	triceps, anconeus, posterior muscles of forearm, skin of the: • posterior aspects of arm and forearm • lateral side of the dorsum of the hand and the dorsal surface of lateral $3^1/_2$ fingers
Medial cord	
medial pectoral nerve (C8, T1)	pectoralis major and minor muscles
medial cutaneous nerve of arm joined (C8, T1)	skin of medial side of arm
medial cutaneous nerve of forearm (C8, T1)	skin of medial side of forearm
ulnar nerve (C8, T1)	flexor carpi ulnaris and medial half of flexor digitorum profundus, hypothenar muscles, adductor pollicis, third and fourth lumbricals, interossei, palmaris brevis, skin of medial half of dorsum of hand and palm, skin of palmar and dorsal surfaces of medial $1^1/_2$ fingers
medial root of median nerve (with lateral root) forms median nerve (C5–C8, T1)	pronator teres, flexor carpi radialis, flexor digitorum superficialis, abductor pollicis brevis, flexor pollicis brevis, opponens pollicis, first two lumbricals (by way of anterior interosseous branch), flexor pollicis longus, flexor digitorum profundus (lateral half), pronator quadratus; palmar cutaneous branch to lateral half of palm and digital branches to palmar surfaces of lateral $3^1/_2$ fingers

Fig. 2.14 Branches of the brachial plexus and their distribution.

21

Axillary lymph nodes

These comprise (Fig. 2.15):

- Lateral group.
- Pectoral group.
- Subscapular group.
- Central group.
- Apical group.

o **Describe the bones and joints of the pectoral region.**
o **Discuss the anatomy of the shoulder joint.**
o **What is the rotator cuff?**
o **List the margins and contents of the axilla.**
o **Describe the brachial plexus.**

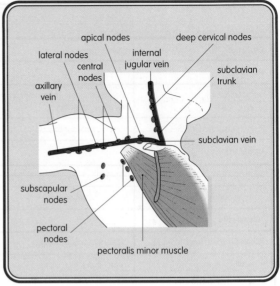

Fig. 2.15 Arrangement of axillary lymph nodes.

THE ARM

The arm lies between the shoulder and elbow joint. It has anterior and posterior compartments separated by the medial and lateral intermuscular septa. These septa arise from the deep fascia surrounding the arm. The lateral intermuscular septum extends from the lateral lip of the intertubercular sulcus to the lateral epicondyle of the humerus. The medial intermuscular septum extends from the medial lip of the intertubercular sulcus to the medial epicondyle of the humerus.

Flexor compartment of the arm

The bony skeleton of the arm and the muscle attachments of the anterior compartment are shown in Fig. 2.16.

Muscles of the arm

The muscles of the arm are shown in Fig. 2.17.

Vessels of the arm

Brachial artery

This is a continuation of the axillary artery, commencing at the lower border of teres major (Fig. 2.18). It terminates at the neck of the radius by dividing into the

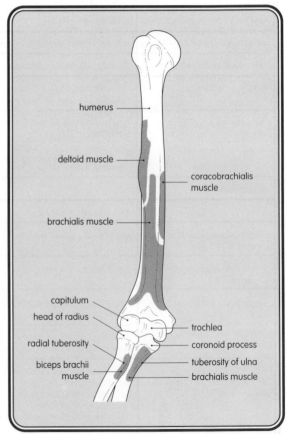

Fig. 2.16 Skeleton of the arm, showing sites of muscle attachment.

Muscles of the upper arm			
Name of muscle (nerve supply)	Origin	Insertion	Action
Anterior fascial compartment			
biceps brachii—long head (musculocutaneous nerve)	supraglenoid tubercle of scapula	tuberosity of radius and bicipital aponeurosis into deep fascia of forearm	supinator of forearm, flexor of elbow joint, weak flexor of shoulder joint
biceps brachii—short head (musculocutaneous nerve)	coracoid process of scapula	tuberosity of radius and bicipital aponeurosis into deep fascia of forearm	supinator of forearm, flexor of elbow joint, weak flexor of shoulder joint
coracobrachialis (musculocutaneous nerve)	coracoid process of scapula	shaft of humerus	flexes and adducts shoulder joint
brachialis (musculocutaneous nerve and radial nerve)	front of humerus	coronoid process of ulna	flexes elbow joint
Posterior fascial compartment			
triceps—long head (radial nerve)	infraglenoid tubercle of scapula	olecranon process of ulna	extends elbow joint
triceps—lateral head (radial nerve)	posterior surface of humerus (upper part)	olecranon process of ulna	extends elbow joint
triceps—medial head (radial nerve)	posterior surface of humerus (lower part)	olecranon process of ulna	extends elbow joint

Fig. 2.17 Muscles of the upper arm. (Adapted from *Clinical Anatomy, An Illustrated Review with Questions and Explanations 2e*, by R.S. Snell. Courtesy of Churchill Livingstone.)

radial and ulnar arteries. The artery is very superficial throughout its course, being covered by skin and fascia only. It lies just behind the medial border of biceps brachii.

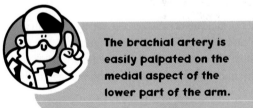

The brachial artery is easily palpated on the medial aspect of the lower part of the arm.

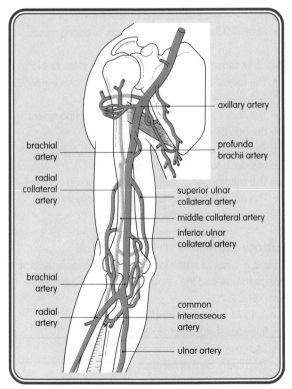

Fig. 2.18 Brachial artery and its branches.

Brachial veins

Usually a pair of venae comitantes accompany the brachial artery. They are joined by tributaries that correspond to branches of the brachial arteries. The veins receive the basilic vein before becoming the axillary vein.

Nerves of the arm

Median nerve

This enters the arm on the lateral side of the brachial artery and crosses in front of the artery to be on its medial side. It continues to the elbow in this relationship and is crossed by the bicipital aponeurosis. The median nerve has no branches in the arm.

Ulnar nerve

This passes down the arm medial to the brachial artery and pierces the medial intermuscular septum halfway down, accompanied by the superior ulnar collateral artery, to enter the posterior compartment. It continues between the medial intermuscular septum and the medial head of triceps, then on the posterior aspect of the medial epicondyle of the humerus, and enters the forearm between the heads of flexor carpi ulnaris muscle. Pressure on the nerve as it crosses the medial epicondyle results in a tingling sensation—this area is referred to as the 'funny bone'. The ulnar nerve has no branches in the arm.

Radial nerve

This enters the posterior compartment of the arm by passing over the lower border of teres major through the triangular interval (see Axilla, p. 19). It runs, with the profunda brachii artery, in the spiral groove of the humerus. The nerve enters the anterior compartment of the arm and then passes into the forearm, deep to the brachioradialis muscle.

Branches in the axilla and arm comprise muscular branches to the triceps and anconeus, and the posterior cutaneous nerve of the arm, the lower lateral cutaneous nerve of the arm, and the posterior cutaneous nerve of the forearm.

Branches at the level of the elbow joint comprise muscular branches to the lateral fibres of brachioradialis and extensor carpi radialis longus.

Musculocutaneous nerve

After its formation, the nerve passes through coracobrachialis and runs down between biceps and brachialis to reach the lateral aspect of brachialis. It supplies the muscles of the anterior compartment and terminates by piercing the deep fascia to become the lateral cutaneous nerve of the forearm.

○ **Describe the vessels, nerves, and muscles of the arm.**

THE CUBITAL FOSSA AND ELBOW JOINT

Cubital fossa

This is a triangular region lying anterior to the elbow joint. Its boundaries are:
- Lateral—brachioradialis muscle.
- Medial—pronator teres.
- Base—an imaginary line drawn between the two epicondyles of the humerus.
- Floor—the supinator and brachialis muscles.
- Roof—skin, fascia, and the bicipital aponeurosis.

Fig. 2.19 shows the contents of the cubital fossa. Note:
- The lateral cutaneous nerve of the forearm emerges between biceps and brachialis.
- The radial nerve enters the anterior compartment deep to brachioradialis.
- The brachial artery crosses the tendon of biceps and lies deep to the bicipital aponeurosis.
- The medial nerve lies medial to the brachial artery.
- The medial cutaneous nerve of the forearm lies superficial to pronator teres.

Elbow joint

This is a synovial hinge joint between the lower end of the humerus and the upper end of the radius and the ulna (Fig. 2.20).

Articular surfaces comprise:
- Superior surface of the radius.
- Capitulum of the humerus laterally.
- Trochlear notch of the ulna.
- Trochlea of the humerus medially.

Movements of the elbow joint are limited to flexion and extension. Independent rotation of the radius is possible at the proximal radioulnar joint in the movements of pronation and supination of the forearm.

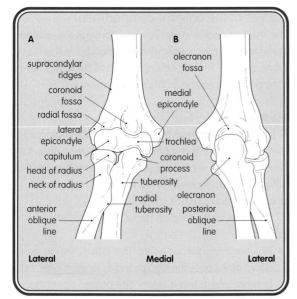

Fig. 2.19 Contents of the cubital fossa.

Fig. 2.20 Anterior (A) and posterior (B) aspects of the humerus and the upper end of the ulna and radius.

The capsule is lax anteroposteriorly, but is strengthened medially and laterally by collateral ligaments.

Ligaments comprise:
- The ulnar collateral ligament—this triangular ligament consists of three bands and runs between the ulnar and humeral bones.
- The radial collateral ligament—this is a band joining the lateral epicondyle of the humerus to the annular ligament.
- The annular ligament—this is attached to the margins of the radial notch of the ulna. It clasps the head and neck of the radius in the proximal radioulnar joint.

The nerve supply of the elbow joint consists of:
- Musculocutaneous nerve.
- Median nerve.
- Ulnar nerve.
- Radial nerve.

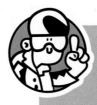

Remember that flexion and extension occur at the elbow joint: rotation occurs at the proximal radioulnar joint.

- List the boundaries and contents of the cubital fossa.
- Describe the elbow joint.

THE FOREARM

The forearm lies between the elbow and wrist joints. It is divided into anterior and posterior compartments by the radius, ulna, and the interosseous membrane (Fig. 2.21). The interosseous membrane is a thin strong membrane uniting the radius and ulnar bones at their interosseous borders. It provides attachments for muscles, and inferiorly it is pierced by the anterior interosseous vessels.

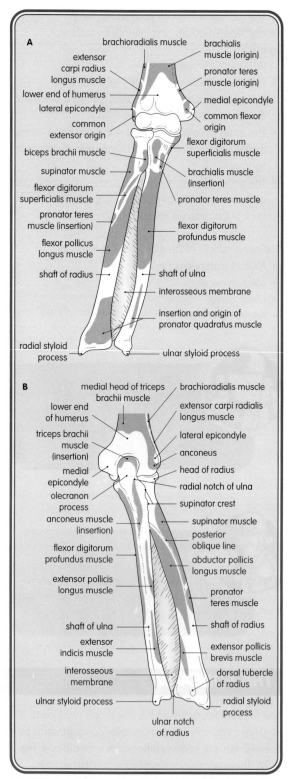

The radial styloid process usually extends more distally than the ulnar styloid process. This relationship is lost in Colles' fracture of the lower end of the radius, where the tips of both processes are level.

Anterior compartment of the forearm

Muscles of the anterior compartment

The muscles of the anterior compartment are divided into superficial and deep groups (Fig. 2.22). The superficial muscles arise from the medial supracondylar ridge and the epicondyle of the humerus, the common flexor origin.

Vessels of the anterior compartment

The brachial artery enters the forearm through the cubital fossa and divides into the radial and ulnar arteries (Fig. 2.23).

Nerves of the anterior compartment

The median and ulnar nerves pass through the anterior compartment and supply all of the muscles in this compartment. The superficial branch of the radial nerve runs part of its course in this compartment.

Median nerve

This enters the forearm between the heads of pronator teres. It crosses the ulnar artery and then runs deep to flexor digitorum superficialis until just above the wrist, where it appears between the tendon of this muscle and the tendon of flexor carpi radialis.

Branches of the median nerve in the forearm comprise:

- Anterior interosseous nerve. This leaves the median nerve as it pases through pronator teres. It joins the anterior interosseous artery and passes down the forearm on the anterior surface of the interosseous membrane between flexor pollicis longus and flexor

Fig. 2.21 Anterior (A) and posterior (B) aspects of the right radius and ulna, showing sites of muscular attachments.

Muscles of the anterior compartment of the forearm			
Name of muscle (nerve supply)	Origin	Insertion	Action
Superficial			
flexor carpi radialis (median nerve)	common flexor origin	second and third metacarpal bones	flexion and abduction of wrist joint
flexor carpi ulnaris—humeral head (ulnar nerve)	common flexor origin	pisiform bone, hook of hamate, base of fifth metacarpal bone	flexion and abduction of wrist joint
flexor carpi ulnaris—ulnar head (ulnar nerve)	olecranon process and posterior border of ulnar	pisiform bone, hook of hamate, base of fifth metacarpal bone	flexion and abduction of wrist joint
flexor digitorum superficialis—humeroulnar head (median nerve)	common flexor origin and ulna	middle phalanges of medial four fingers	flexes middle and proximal phalanges of middle four fingers
flexor digitorum superficialis—radial head (median nerve)	oblique line on anterior surface of radius	middle phalanges of medial four fingers	flexes middle and proximal phalanges of middle four fingers
pronator teres—humeral head (median nerve)	common flexor origin	lateral aspect of shaft of radius	pronation of forearm and flexion of elbow
pronator teres—ulnar head (median nerve)	coronoid process of ulna	lateral aspect of shaft of radius	pronation of forearm
Deep			
pronator quadratus (anterior interosseous nerve)	anterior surface of ulna	anterior surface of radius	pronation of forearm
flexor pollicis longus (anterior interosseous nerve)	anterior surface of radius	distal phalanx of thumb	flexes all of thumb
flexor digitorum profundus (medial half by ulnar nerve and lateral half by median nerve)	anterior surface of ulna, interosseous membrane	distal phalanges of medial four fingers	flexes all of fingers

Fig. 2.22 Muscles of the anterior compartment of the forearm.

digitorum profundus. It supplies flexor pollicis longus, the lateral part of flexor digitorum profundus, and pronator quadratus, and has articular branches to the distal radioulnar, wrist, and carpal joints.
- Muscular branches to the superficial muscles except flexor carpi ulnaris.
- Palmar cutaneous nerve. This is given off just above the wrist joint. It supplies the skin over the thenar eminence and the central part of the palm of the hand.
- Articular branches to the elbow joint and proximal radioulnar joint.

Recognize that the median nerve supplies most of the muscles of the flexor compartment.

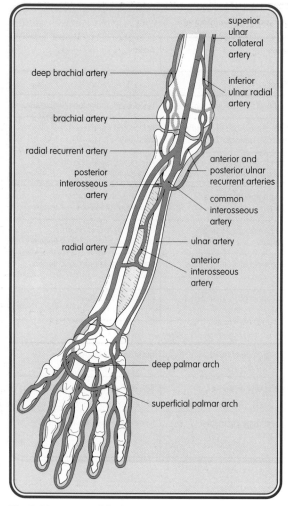

superior ulnar collateral artery

deep brachial artery

inferior ulnar radial artery

brachial artery

radial recurrent artery

posterior interosseous artery

anterior and posterior ulnar recurrent arteries

common interosseous artery

radial artery

ulnar artery

anterior interosseous artery

deep palmar arch

superficial palmar arch

Fig. 2.23 Arteries of the forearm.

Ulnar nerve

This enters the anterior compartment by passing between the heads of flexor carpi ulnaris. It runs with the ulnar artery between flexor carpi ulnaris and flexor digitorum profundus. In the lower half of the forearm both artery and nerve become superficial on the lateral side of flexor carpi ulnaris.

Branches of the ulnar nerve comprise:

- Muscular branches to flexor carpi ulnaris and the medial half of flexor digitorum profundus
- A palmar cutaneous branch, which supplies the skin over the medial part of the palm.

- A dorsal branch, which passes deep to flexor carpi ulnaris to reach the dorsal aspect of the hand.

Radial nerve

This enters the forearm deep to the brachioradialis muscle. It immediately divides into a superficial and a deep branch. The deep branch passes laterally around the radius between the layers of supinator to enter the extensor compartment as the posterior interosseous nerve. The superficial branch continues down the forearm deep to brachioradialis and is joined by the radial artery. Both pass onto the dorsum of the hand.

Posterior compartment of the forearm

Muscles of the posterior compartment

The superficial group of muscles arise from the lateral epicondyle (the common extensor origin) and the supracondylar ridge of the humerus (Fig. 2.24).

Vessels of the posterior compartment

The ulnar artery gives off the common interosseous artery near its origin. The latter divides into the anterior and posterior interosseous arteries, which both contribute to the supply for the extensor compartment.

The anterior interosseous artery passes down the anterior surface of the interosseous membrane. Branches pierce the membrane to supply the underlying muscles. At the superior border of pronator quadratus the artery pierces the membrane to anastomose with the posterior interosseous artery and then continues to the wrist to join the dorsal carpal arch.

The posterior interosseous artery passes posteriorly above the upper border of the interosseous membrane and accompanies the posterior interosseous nerve to supply the deep muscles of the extensor compartment.

Nerves of the posterior compartment

Brachioradialis and extensor carpi radialis longus are supplied directly by the radial nerve. All the other extensor muscles are supplied by the posterior interosseous nerve.

This nerve emerges from supinator and runs on the interosseous membrane as far as the wrist joint, which it supplies.

Muscles of the posterior compartment of the forearm			
Name of muscle (nerve supply)	Origin	Insertion	Action
brachioradialis (radial nerve)	lateral supracondylar ridge of humerus	styloid process of radius	flexes elbow and rotates forearm
extensor carpi radialis longus (radial nerve)	common extensor origin	base of second metacarpal bone	extends and abducts hand at wrist joint
extensor carpi radialis brevis (posterior interosseous nerve)	common extensor origin	base of third metacarpal bone	extends and abducts hand at wrist joint
extensor digitorum (posterior interosseous nerve)		middle and distal phalanges of the medial four fingers	extends fingers, hand and wrist
extensor digiti minimi (posterior interosseous nerve)		extensor expansion of little finger	extends little finger
extensor carpi ulnaris (posterior interosseous nerve)		base of fifth metacarpal bone	extends and adducts hand at the wrist
anconeus (posterior interosseous nerve)		olecranon process of ulna	extends elbow joint
supinator (posterior interosseous nerve)	common extensor origin and ulna	neck and shaft of radius	supination of forearm
abductor pollicis longus (posterior interosseous nerve)	shafts of radius and ulna and interosseous membrane	base of first metacarpal bone	abducts thumb
extensor pollicis brevis (posterior interosseous nerve)	shaft of radius and interosseous membrane	base of proximal phalanx of thumb	extends metacarpophalangeal joint of thumb
extensor pollicis longus (posterior interosseous nerve)	shafts of ulna and interosseous membrane	base of distal phalanx of thumb	extends thumb
extensor indicis (posterior interossoeus nerve)		extensor expansion of index finger	extends index finger

Fig. 2.24 Muscles of the posterior compartment of the forearm.

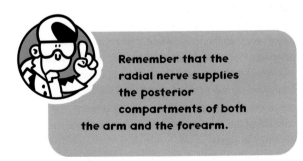

Remember that the radial nerve supplies the posterior compartments of both the arm and the forearm.

Anatomical snuffbox

This is a depression proximal to the base of the first metacarpal and overlying the scaphoid and trapezoid bones when the thumb is actively extended. The anterior margin is formed by the tendons of abductor pollicis longus and extensor pollicis brevis. The posterior margin is formed by the tendon of extensor pollicis longus. The radial artery runs through the anatomical snuffbox on its course to the dorsum of the hand. It lies on the scaphoid bone here.

Acute tenderness in this region following a fall indicates possible fracture of the scaphoid bone.

Radioulnar joints

The movements of pronation and supination occur at the proximal and distal radioulnar joints. In the proximal radioulnar joint, the head of radius rotates in an osseofibrous ring formed by the radial notch of the ulna and the annular ligament. The radius also rotates around the ulna in the distal radioulnar joint.

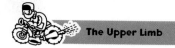

Biceps brachii and supinator cause supination, whereas pronator teres and quadratus are responsible for pronation.

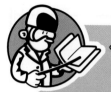

° **List the muscles, nerves, and vessels of the anterior compartment of the forearm.**

° **Describe the muscles, nerves, and vessels of the posterior compartment of the forearm.**

° **Outline the boundaries and contents of the anatomical snuffbox.**

THE WRIST AND HAND

Fig. 2.25 shows the skeleton of the wrist and hand.

Wrist (radiocarpal) joint

This is a synovial joint where the distal end of the radius articulates with the scaphoid, lunate, and triquetral bones. An articular disc separates the joint cavity from the distal radioulnar joint (Fig. 2.26).

Movements of the wrist joint are inseparable functionally from those at the midcarpal joint (synovial joints between the proximal and distal rows of carpal bones):

• The midcarpal joint participates mainly in flexion and abduction.

• The radiocarpal joint contributes mainly to extension and adduction.

All the joints in the wrist and hand are synovial joints.

Dorsum of the hand

The skin on the dorsum of the hand is thin and loose and the dorsal venous network of veins is usually visible. The veins drain into the cephalic and basilic veins.

The long extensor tendons of the forearm lie beneath the superficial veins. As the tendons cross the wrist joint, they are surrounded by synovial sheaths and bound down by the extensor retinaculum. The dorsal interossei are the only intrinsic muscles of the dorsum of the hand. Dorsal digital expansions are the expanded tendons of the extensor digitorum (Fig. 2.27).

Nerve supply to the dorsum of the hand

Fig. 2.28 shows the cutaneous innervation of the hand. Note the fingertips are supplied by palmar digital branches of the median and ulnar nerves.

Vessels of the dorsum of the hand

Fig. 2.29 shows the blood supply to the dorsum of the hand.

Palm of the hand

Skin

The skin is thick and hairless. Flexure creases and papillary ridges occupy the entire flexor surface and improve the gripping ability of the hand. Fibrous bands bind the skin down to the palmar aponeurosis and divide the subcutaneous fat into loculi, forming a cushion capable of withstanding pressure.

Palmar aponeurosis

This is a tough sheet lying between the thenar and hypothenar eminences, where it is continuous with the deep fascia. Distally it separates into four slips, which are joined by the superficial transverse metacarpal ligaments. At the base of each finger the four slips divide and fuse with the fibrous flexor sheaths, the capsule of the metacarpophalangeal joint, and the proximal phalanx.

Contraction of the palmar aponeurosis leads to fixed flexion of the digits (Dupuytren's contracture), which affects most severely the ring and little fingers.

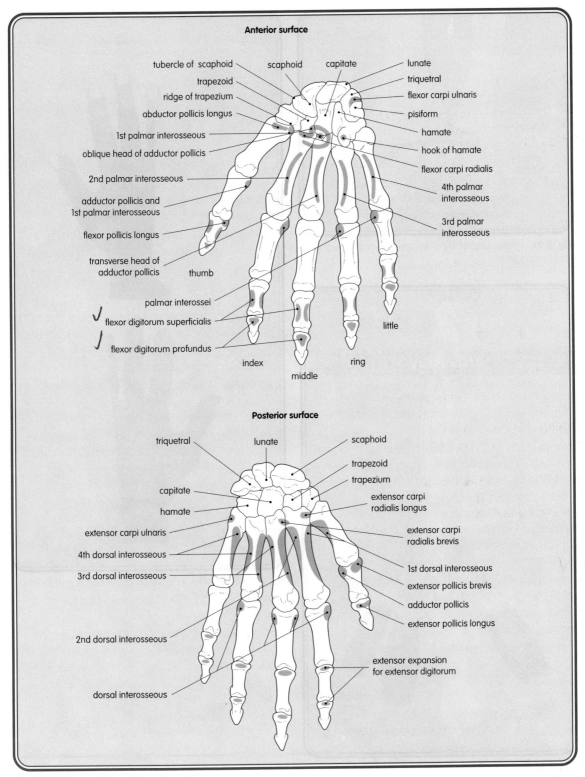

Fig. 2.25 Bones of the wrist and hand.

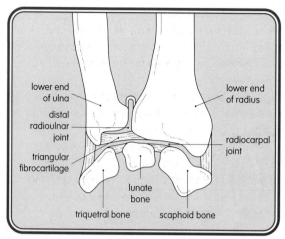

Fig. 2.26 Relationship of the distal radioulnar joint to the radiocarpal joint.

lower end of ulna

distal radioulnar joint

triangular fibrocartilage

triquetral bone

lunate bone

scaphoid bone

lower end of radius

radiocarpal joint

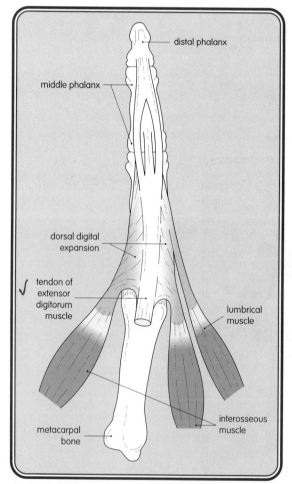

distal phalanx

middle phalanx

dorsal digital expansion

✓ tendon of extensor digitorum muscle

lumbrical muscle

interosseous muscle

metacarpal bone

Fig. 2.27 Dorsal digital expansion and extensor tendon.

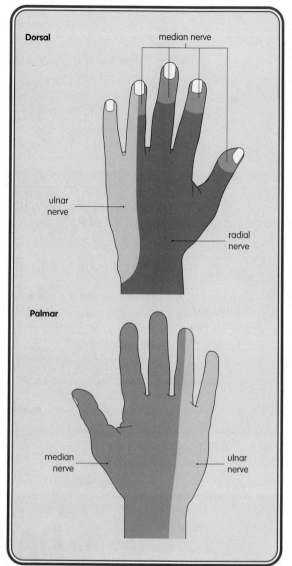

Dorsal

median nerve

ulnar nerve

radial nerve

Palmar

median nerve

ulnar nerve

Fig. 2.28 Cutaneous innervation of the dorsal and palmar surfaces of the hand.

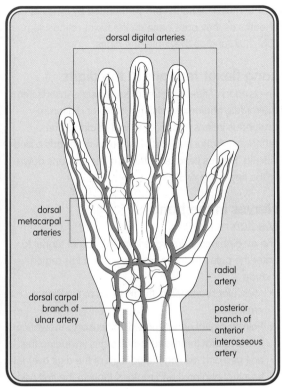

dorsal digital arteries

dorsal metacarpal arteries

dorsal carpal branch of ulnar artery

radial artery

posterior branch of anterior interosseous artery

Fig. 2.29 Vessels of the dorsum of the hand.

Flexor retinaculum

This strong band runs from the scaphoid and trapezium to the pisiform and hook of the hamate. It forms an osseofibrous canal with the carpal bones, the carpal tunnel (Fig. 2.30).

The muscles of the thenar and hypothenar eminences arise from the flexor retinaculum and adjacent carpal bones.

Compression of the median nerve in the carpal tunnel results in wasting of the thenar muscles and anaesthesia of the lateral three-and-a-half digits. This is known as carpal tunnel syndrome. Division of the retinaculum relieves the pressure and symptoms.

Fig. 2.30 Cross-section of the carpal tunnel and its contents.

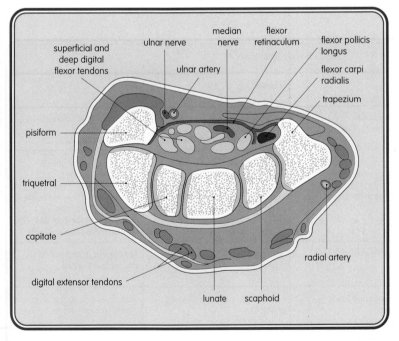

superficial and deep digital flexor tendons

ulnar nerve

median nerve

flexor retinaculum

flexor pollicis longus

ulnar artery

flexor carpi radialis

trapezium

pisiform

triquetral

capitate

radial artery

digital extensor tendons

lunate

scaphoid

Muscles of the hand
Thenar eminence
This is the prominent region between the base of the thumb and the wrist. It is composed of three muscles: abductor pollicis brevis, flexor pollicis brevis, and opponens pollicis (Fig. 2.31).

Hypothenar eminence
This lies between the base of the small finger and the wrist. It consists of the abductor digiti minimi, flexor digiti minimi, and opponens digiti minimi. These, and other small muscles of the hand, are discussed in Fig. 2.31.

The median nerve supplies the thenar eminence; the ulnar nerve supplies the hypothenar eminence.

Long flexor tendons in the hand
The following flexor tendons enter the hand: flexor carpi ulnaris, flexor carpi radialis, flexor digitorum superficialis and profundus, and flexor pollicis longus.

The muscle tendons are surrounded by synovial sheaths as they pass beneath the flexor retinaculum (Fig. 2.32) and as they enter the digits.

Long flexor tendons in the digits
The tendon of flexor digitorum superficialis inserts into the middle phalanx, whilst that of flexor digitorum profundus inserts into the terminal phalanx. The tendons are attached to their sheaths via bands called vincula. Fibrous flexor sheaths bind the tendons down to the finger (Fig. 2.33).

Nerves in the hand
Median nerve
The median nerve emerges from the carpal tunnel to enter the palm. Branches of the nerve in this region include:

- Muscular branches to the muscles of the thenar eminence.
- Palmar digital nerves providing sensory innervation to the lateral three-and-a-half digits (including the nail bed and skin on the dorsum of the digit over the terminal phalanx) and motor supply to the first and second lumbricals.

Small muscles of the hand			
Name of muscle (nerve supply)	Origin	Insertion	Action
lumbricals (first and second: median nerve; third and fourth: ulnar nerve)	tendons of flexor digitorum profundus	extensor expansion of medial four fingers	flex metacarpophalangeal joints and extend interphalangeal joints
interossei—palmar (deep branch of ulnar nerve; first to fourth)	first, second, fourth, and fifth metacarpal bones	base of proximal phalanges and extensor expansion	adduct fingers and thumb towards the centre
interossei—dorsal (deep branch of ulnar nerve; first to fourth)	sides of five metacarpal bones	base of proximal phalanges and extensor expansion	abduct fingers from the centre; all interossei also flex metacarpophalangeal and extend interphalangeal joints
hypothenar—abductor, flexor, and opponens digiti minimi (deep branch of ulnar nerve)	flexor retinaculum	little finger	flex little finger and pull fifth metacarpal forward
thenar—abductor pollicis brevis, flexor pollicis brevis, opponens pollicis (median nerve):	carpal bones and flexor retinaculum	phalanx and metacarpal bones of thumb	abduct, flex, adduct, and move thumb medially across the palm
adductor pollicis (deep branch of ulnar nerve)	carpal bones and flexor retinaculum	phalanx and metacarpal bones of thumb	abduct, flex, adduct, and move thumb medially across the palm

Fig. 2.31 Small muscles of the hand.

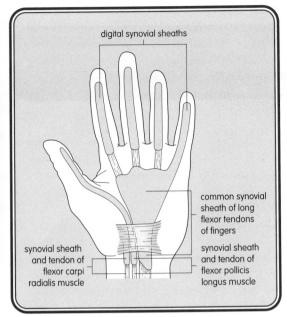

Fig. 2.32 Flexor synovial sheaths in the hand.

Labels on figure:
- digital synovial sheaths
- common synovial sheath of long flexor tendons of fingers
- synovial sheath and tendon of flexor carpi radialis muscle
- synovial sheath and tendon of flexor pollicis longus muscle

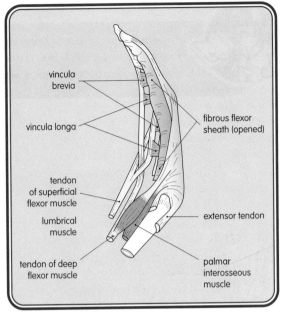

Fig. 2.33 Long flexor tendons of a finger and their vincula.

Labels on figure:
- vincula brevia
- vincula longa
- tendon of superficial flexor muscle
- lumbrical muscle
- tendon of deep flexor muscle
- fibrous flexor sheath (opened)
- extensor tendon
- palmar interosseous muscle

Ulnar nerve

The ulnar nerve and artery pass into the hand together, superficial to the flexor retinaculum. The nerve divides into superficial and deep branches:

- The superficial branch supplies palmaris brevis and a palmar digital nerves to the medial one-and-a-half digits (including the skin over the dorsum of the distal phalanx).
- The deep branch runs with the deep branch of the ulnar artery and supplies the hypothenar muscles, the medial lumbricals, the interosseous muscles, adductor pollicis.

> **Damage to the median nerve, e.g. trauma to the wrist, results in loss of sensation to the lateral three-and-a-half digits and loss of function in the thumb. This is a very incapacitating injury and renders the entire upper limb almost functionless.**

See Fig. 2.28 for the cutaneous innervation of the palmar and dorsal surfaces of the hand.

Vessels of the hand

The radial artery slopes across the anatomical snuffbox overlying the scaphoid and trapezium and passes into the hand between the two heads of the first dorsal interosseous.

The ulnar artery approaches the wrist between flexor digitorum superficialis and flexor carpi ulnaris. It enters the wrist with the ulnar nerve, superficial to the flexor retinaculum.

Palmar spaces

The intermediate palmar septum from the palmar aponeurosis to the third metacarpal divides the central part of the palm into two fascial spaces: the thenar space lies laterally and the midpalmar space lies medially.

The spaces communicate with the subcutaneous tissue of the webs of the fingers. Deep infections of the midpalmar space often spread to these sites.

Nails

These lie on the dorsal surface of the distal phalanges and are formed from modified skin tissue.

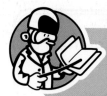

○ Describe a dorsal digital expansion.
○ List the muscles, vessels, and nerves of the palm of the hand.
○ Outline the carpal tunnel and the structures passing through it.

3. The Thorax

REGIONS AND COMPONENTS OF THE THORAX

The thorax lies between the neck and the abdomen.

The thoracic cavity contains the heart, lungs, great vessels, trachea, and oesophagus. The lungs lie laterally and the other structures lie in the mediastinum.

The thoracic cage is formed by the thoracic vertebrae, the ribs, the costal cartilages, and the sternum. It protects the contents of the thoracic cavity and some abdominal contents, e.g. the liver and spleen.

Superiorly the thorax communicates with the neck through the thoracic inlet. Inferiorly the diaphragm separates the thorax from the abdominal cavity.

SURFACE ANATOMY AND SUPERFICIAL STRUCTURES

Bony landmarks

The bony landmarks of the thorax are illustrated in Fig. 3.1.

The bony sternum can be palpated in the midline of the thorax anteriorly. The manubrium sterni joins the body of the sternum at the manubriosternal joint (the angle of Louis). The manubriosternal angle is important clinically as it is level with the second costal cartilage. Inferiorly the body of the sternum articulates with the xiphoid process.

Ribs 1–6 articulate with the manubrium and sternum laterally via the costal cartilages. The costal margin runs from the xiphisternum and comprises the costal cartilages of ribs 7–10.

Posteriorly the spinous processes of the thoracic vertebrae are palpable inferior to the vertebra prominens—the spinous process of C7 vertebra.

Trachea, lungs, and pleurae

The trachea is palpable in the midline, above the suprasternal notch.

The dome of the pleura extends about 2.5 cm above the medial end of the clavicle (Fig. 3.2). The anterior border of the right pleura passes down behind the sternal angle to the xiphisternal joint. The

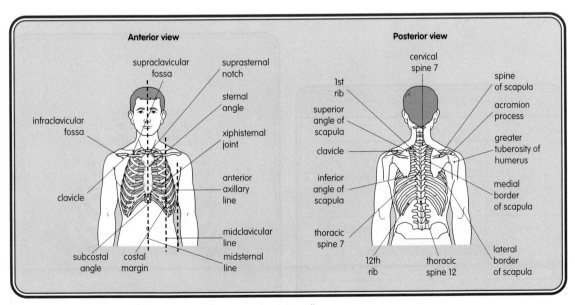

Fig. 3.1 Surface markings of the anterior and posterior thoracic walls.

anterior border of the left pleura follows a similar course, but at the level of the 4th costal cartilage it deviates laterally to form the cardiac notch. The lower border follows a curved line, being at the level of the 8th rib in the midclavicular line, the 10th rib in the midaxillary line, and the 12th rib adjacent to the vertebral column.

Note, trauma to the root of the neck or at the 11th or 12th ribs can easily penetrate the pleura, causing a pneumothorax.

The surface markings of the lungs in mid-inspiration are similar to those of the pleurae except inferiorly, where it lies at the level of the 6th, 8th, and 10th ribs in the midclavicular line, midaxillary line, and adjacent to the vertebral column, respectively.

The space between the lower border of the pleura and lung is the costodiaphragmatic recess. In life it is filled by the lungs in full inspiration.

Heart

The surface markings of the heart are outlined in Fig. 3.3. The surface markings of the heart valves are illustrated in Fig. 3.4.

Great vessels

The aortic arch, the roots of the brachiocephalic and left common carotid and subclavian arteries, the superior vena cava and its tributaries, and the brachiocephalic veins all lie behind the manubrium.

The internal thoracic vessels run vertically downwards, posterior to the costal cartilages and 1 cm lateral to the sternal edge, as far as the 6th intercostal space.

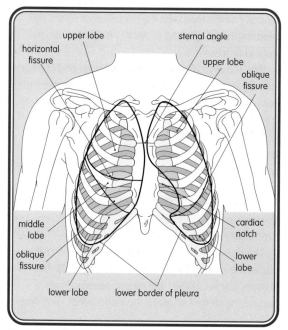

Fig. 3.2 Surface markings of the lungs and pleurae.

Outline of the surface landmarks of the heart	
Border	**Area covered**
superior border	from the second left costal cartilage to the third right costal cartilage
right border	from the third right costal cartilage to the sixth right costal cartilage
left border	from the second left costal cartilage to the apex of the heart
inferior border	from the sixth right costal cartilage to the apex
apex	lies in the fifth intercostal space, about 9 cm from the midline

Fig. 3.3 Outline of the surface landmarks of the heart.

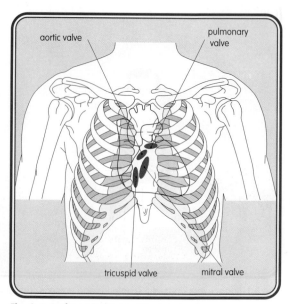

Fig. 3.4 Surface markings of the heart valves.

Diaphragm

The central tendon of the diaphragm lies behind the xiphisternal joint. In mid-respiration the right dome arches upwards to the upper border of the 5th rib in the midclavicular line; the left dome reaches only the lower border of the 5th rib.

Breasts

The breasts lie in the superficial fascia, mainly superficial to the pectoralis major muscle. They contain mammary glands, which drain by lactiferous ducts into the nipple. The nipple is the greatest prominence of the breast and is surrounded by a circular pigmented area called the areola.

The base of the breast usually lies between the 2nd and 6th rib vertically, and from the midaxillary line to the lateral border of the sternum horizontally.

The blood supply to the breast is derived from branches of the internal thoracic artery, the lateral thoracic and the thoracoacromial arteries, and the posterior intercostal arteries. Venous drainage is into the axillary and internal thoracic veins.

Lymph drains into the subareolar plexus and then into either axillary nodes or supraclavicular and infraclavicular nodes.

Axillary nodes receive most of the lymphatic drainage of the superior and lateral parts of the breast. Lymphatics from the inferior and medial part of the breast drain into lymph nodes along the internal thoracic vessels and then via the broncho mediastinal lymph trunk into the lymphatics at the root of the neck (supra- and infraclavicular nodes).

Lymphatics may communicate with vessels from the opposite breast.

Carcinoma of the breast—the most common cancer affecting women—spreads via the lymphatics in many cases. A detailed knowledge of this drainage is required for appropriate treatment.

○ **Describe the structure, blood supply, and lymphatic drainage of the breast.**
○ **Outline the surface anatomy of the heart, lungs, and pleura.**

THE THORACIC WALL

The thoracic skeleton is formed by the sternum, the ribs and costal cartilages, and the thoracic vertebrae (Fig. 3.5).

Sternum

The sternum (breast bone) has three components:
- The manubrium is the upper part of the sternum. It articulates with the clavicles and with the 1st and upper part of the 2nd costal cartilages.
- The body of the sternum articulates with the manubrium at the manubriosternal joint superiorly, and with the xiphisternum inferiorly. These are fibrocartilaginous joints. Laterally the sternal body articulates with the 2nd to 7th costal cartilages via synovial joints.
- The xiphoid process is the lowest part of the sternum.

Ribs and costal cartilages

There are 12 pairs of ribs. They all articulate with a costal cartilage medially. The upper seven ribs articulate directly with the sternum via their own costal cartilage. The 8th to 10th ribs have costal cartilages that are attached to each other and to the 7th anteriorly, and thence to the sternum.

The floating 11th and 12th ribs have no anterior attachment for their costal cartilages.

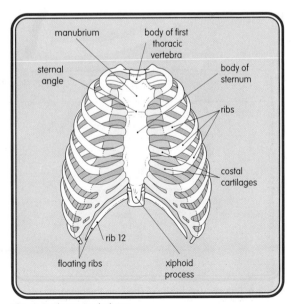

Fig. 3.5 Thoracic skeleton.

Typical ribs

A typical rib has the following features (Fig. 3.6):

- It is a long curved flattened bone with a rounded superior border and a sharp thin inferior border forming the costal groove.
- It has a head with two demifacets for articulation with the numerically similar vertebral body and that of the vertebra immediately above.
- The neck separates the head and the tubercle.
- The tubercle has a facet for articulation with the transverse process of the corresponding vertebra.
- The shaft is thin, flat, and curved, with an angle at its point of greatest change in curvature.

Atypical ribs

Fig. 3.7 shows the 1st rib and its relations in the thoracic inlet. This is the broadest, shortest, and most sharply curved rib. It has a tubercle on the medial surface for attachment of the scalenus anterior. The subclavian artery and vein pass posterior and anterior to the tubercle, respectively. The artery forms the subclavian groove on the rib.

The 10th, 11th, and 12th ribs have one facet on the head for articulation with their own vertebra.

A cervical rib may compress the subclavian artery or the inferior trunk of the brachial plexus, causing ischaemic pain and numbness along the medial border of the forearm.

Thoracic vertebrae

There are 12 thoracic vertebrae with their intervening intervertebral discs (Fig. 3.8).

Openings into the thorax
Thoracic inlet

The thoracic cavity communicates with the root of the neck via the thoracic inlet (see Fig. 3.7). The margins of the inlet include:

- T1 vertebra.
- Medial border of the 1st rib and its costal cartilage.
- Superior border of the manubrium.

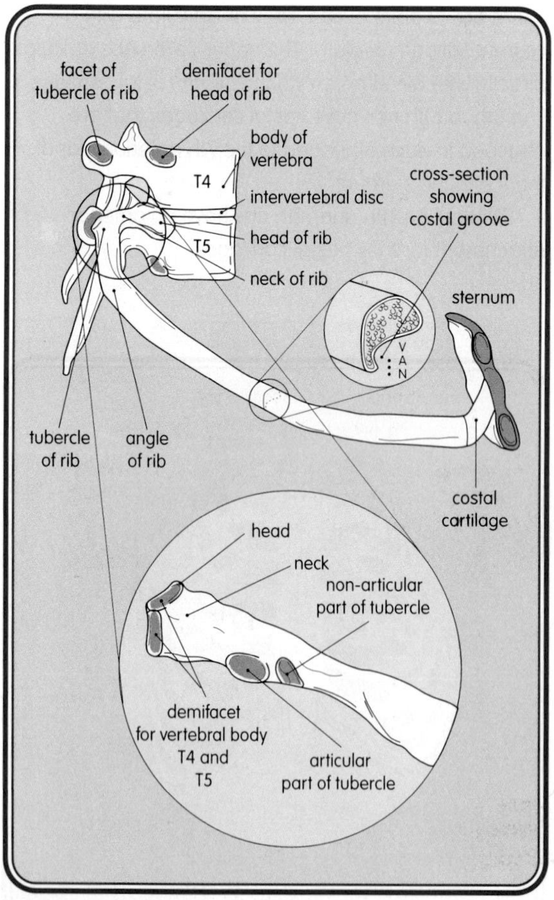

Fig. 3.6 Fifth rib, with the inset showing the posterior surface of the rib.

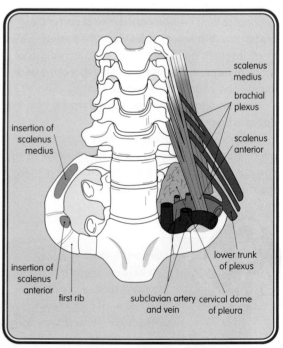

Fig. 3.7 First rib and its relations to the thoracic inlet.

The oesophagus, trachea, and the apices of the lungs, together with various vessels and nerves, pass through the inlet.

Thoracic outlet
This lies between the thorax and the abdomen and is covered mainly by the diaphragm. Numerous structures pass through this opening (see Fig. 3.12).

Intercostal spaces
The intercostal spaces lie between the ribs.

Below the skin and superficial fascia lie the three intercostal muscles (Fig. 3.9). The innermost muscle

layer is lined by the endothoracic fascia and the parietal pleura.

Fig. 3.9 outlines the muscles of the thorax.

Intercostal nerves and vessels
The intercostal nerves are the anterior rami of the upper thoracic spinal nerves. The 12th nerve is the subcostal nerve.

Each intercostal nerve runs in a plane between the parietal pleura and the posterior intercostal membrane and passes forward in the costal groove of the corresponding rib, between the two deeper intercostal muscles.

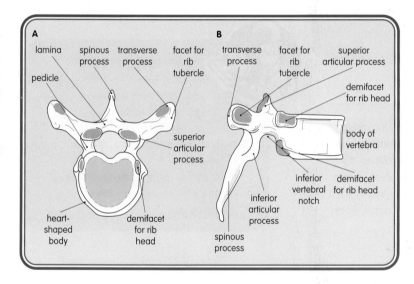

Fig. 3.8 Superior (A) and lateral (B) surfaces of a thoracic vertebra.

Muscles of the thorax			
Name of muscle (nerve supply)	Origin	Insertion	Action
external intercostal (intercostal)	inferior border of rib above	superior border of rib above	all the intercostal muscles assist in both inspiration and expiration during ventilation
internal intercostal (intercostal)	inferior border of rib above	superior border of rib above	
innermost intercostal (intercostal)	adjacent ribs	adjacent ribs	
diaphragm (phrenic)	xiphoid process, lower sixth costal cartilages, L1–L3 vertebrae by crura, and medial and lateral arcuate ligaments	central tendon	important muscle of inspiration; increases vertical diameter of thorax by pulling down central tendon

Fig. 3.9 Muscles of the thorax.

All the intercostal nerves supply the skin and parietal pleura and the intercostal muscles of their respective spaces. Most of the first intercostal nerve passes to the brachial plexus. The 7th to 11th nerves also pass to the anterior abdominal wall to supply the skin, peritoneum, and anterior abdominal wall muscles. The subcostal nerve lies in the abdominal wall.

Fig. 3.10 shows the arterial supply to the thoracic wall.

The position of the vessels and nerves in the intercostal space is always vein, artery, nerve (VAN) from above downwards.

Diaphragm

This is the primary muscle of respiration. It consists of a peripheral muscular part and a central tendon, and separates the thoracic and abdominal cavities. As viewed from the front, the diaphragm curves up into two domes, the right dome being higher than the left (Fig. 3.11). When viewed from the side, it assumes an inverted-J shape.

Fig. 3.12 lists the openings in the diaphragm and the structures passing through them.

The blood and nerve supplies of the diaphragm are shown in Fig. 3.13.

The phrenic nerve is the sole motor supply to the diaphragm.

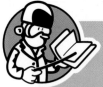

- Describe the bones of the thoracic wall.
- Describe a typical intercostal space.
- List the intercostal nerves and vessels.
- Outline the diaphragm and the structures passing through it.

Arterial supply to the thoracic wall		
Artery	Origin	Distribution
anterior intercostal (spaces 1–6)	internal thoracic artery	intercostal spaces and parietal pleura
anterior intercostal (spaces 7–9)	musculophrenic artery	
posterior intercostal (spaces 1–2)	superior intercostal artery	
posterior intercostal (all other spaces)	thoracic aorta	
internal thoracic	subclavian artery	runs down lateral to the sternum and terminates by dividing into the superior epigastric and musculophrenic arteries
subcostal	thoracic aorta	abdominal wall

Fig. 3.10 Arterial supply to the thoracic wall.

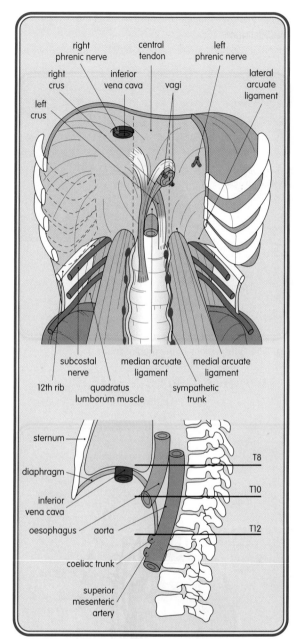

Fig. 3.11 Diaphragm as seen from below and as a sagittal section (the anterior portion of the right side has been removed).

Diaphragmatic apertures and structures passing through them	
Opening	**Structures**
aortic opening (level of T12)	aorta, thoracic duct, azygos vein
oesophageal opening (level of T10)	oesophagus, vagus nerves, oesophageal branches of the gastric vessels and lymphatics
vena caval opening (level of T8 in the central tendon)	inferior vena cava, right phrenic nerve
other structures passing through the diaphragm	greater, lesser, and least splanchnic nerves; sympathetic trunk; left phrenic nerve; neurovascular bundles of the 7th to 12th intercostal nerves; superior epigastric artery

Fig. 3.12 Diaphragmatic apertures and structures passing through them.

Nerves and vessels of the diaphragm	
innervation	motor supply: phrenic nerves (C3–C5); sensory supply: centrally by phrenic nerves (C3–C5), peripherally by intercostal nerves (T5–T11) and subcostal nerve (T12)
arterial supply	superior phrenic arteries; musculophrenic arteries; inferior phrenic arteries
venous drainage	musculophrenic and pericardiacophrenic veins drain into internal thoracic vein; inferior phrenic veins
lymphatic drainage	diaphragmatic lymph nodes drain to posterior mediastinal nodes eventually; superior lumbar lymph nodes; lymphatic plexuses on superior and inferior surfaces communicate freely

Fig. 3.13 Nerves and vessels of the diaphragm.

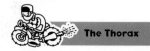

THE THORACIC CAVITY

The thoracic cavity is filled laterally by the lungs and the pleural cavities. The median partition separating the lungs and pleurae is the mediastinum. This may be divided by a plane passing through the sternal angle (of Louis) and T4 vertebra (Fig. 3.14). The superior mediastinum lies above this plane and contains the thymus, great vessels, trachea, oesophagus, thoracic duct, and sympathetic trunk. The inferior mediastinum lies below the plane and is further subdivided:

- The anterior mediastinum, lying between the pericardium and the sternum, contains lymph nodes.
- The middle mediastinum contains the pericardium and heart.
- The posterior mediastinum, lying between the pericardium and the vertebral column, contains the oesophagus, thoracic duct, sympathetic trunk, and descending aorta.

Fig. 3.15 shows the left and right sides of the mediastinum.

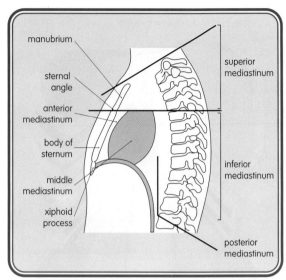

Fig. 3.14 Subdivisions of the mediastinum.

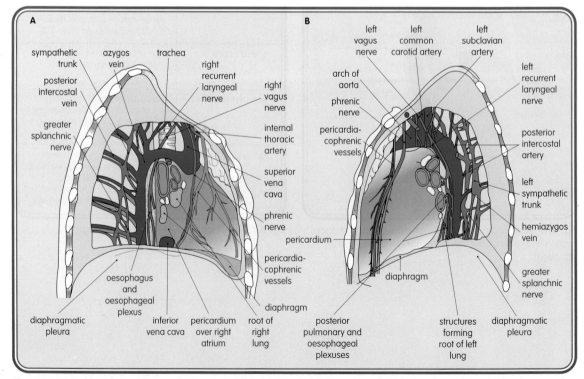

Fig. 3.15 (A) Right surface of the mediastinum and the right posterior thoracic wall. (B) Left surface of the mediastinum and the left posterior thoracic wall. Mediastinal pleura has been removed.

THE MEDIASTINUM

Pericardium

This is a double-walled fibroserous sac that encloses the heart and the roots of the great vessels. It is divided into the fibrous pericardium and the two layers of the serous pericardium: parietal and visceral. The fibrous pericardium is a strong layer that limits the movement of the heart. It is attached to the central tendon of the diaphragm, the sternum, and the tunica adventitia of the great vessels.

The pericardium may be affected in many diseases, including tuberculosis and other infections. Also, trauma to the heart may result in bleeding into the pericardium, which may compress the heart (cardiac tamponade) and is an emergency—immediate drainage is needed if the patient is to survive.

Pericardial sinuses

The reflection of the serous pericardium around the large veins forms a recess called the oblique sinus. The reflection around the aorta and the pulmonary trunk, together with the reflection around the great veins, form the transverse sinus. Both sinuses lie on the posterior surface of the heart.

Heart

This is the muscular organ responsible for pumping blood throughout the body (Fig. 3.16). It lies free in the pericardium, connected only at its base to the great vessels.

The walls of the heart consist mainly of heart muscle (myocardium), lined internally by the endocardium and externally by the epicardium (visceral serous pericardium).

The heart has four chambers: two atria and two ventricles. The right side of the heart pumps blood to the lungs while the left side propels blood throughout the remainder of the body.

Chambers of the heart
Right atrium

This chamber consists of the right atrium proper and an atrial appendage, the right auricle (Fig. 3.17). The two parts are separated externally by a groove—the sulcus terminalis—and internally by a ridge—the crista terminalis. The area posterior to the crista terminalis is smooth walled, while the region anterior to it is ridged by muscle fibres, the musculi pectinati.

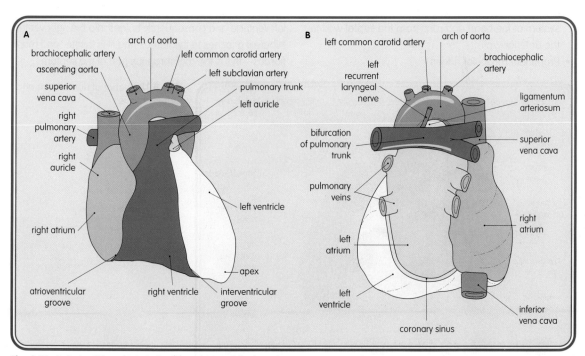

Fig. 3.16 Anterior (A) and posterior (B) surfaces of the heart.

Interatrial septum

This forms the posterior wall of the right atrium. In the lower part of the septum is a depression, the fossa ovalis. This represents the foramen ovale in the foetal heart. The annulus ovalis forms the crescentic upper margin of the fossa. It is the remnant of the lower edge of the septum secundum of the foetal heart.

Right ventricle

This chamber communicates with the right atrium via the tricuspid valve (see Fig. 3.17) and with the pulmonary artery through the pulmonary valve. The ventricle becomes funnel shaped as it approaches the pulmonary orifice—this region is known as the infundibulum.

The tricuspid valve has three cusps (anterior, posterior, and septal), the bases of which are attached to the fibrous ring of the skeleton of the heart.

The three cusps of the pulmonary valve are attached to the arterial wall at their lower margins. At the root of the pulmonary trunk are three dilations called the sinuses, one external to each cusp.

The ventricular wall has many muscular elevations, called trabeculae carneae, of which there are three types:

- Papillary muscles—attached to the ventricular wall and to the cusps of the tricuspid valve via fibrous cords, the chordae tendineae.
- Moderator band—forms part of the conducting system of the heart and runs from the septal wall to the anterior wall.
- Prominent muscular ridges.

Left atrium

This consists of a main cavity and an atrial appendage, the left auricle. The interior is smooth, but the auricle is ridged. The left atrium forms most of the base of the heart. The four pulmonary veins open into the posterior wall. The left atrioventricular orifice is protected by the bicuspid mitral valve.

Left ventricle

The left ventricle is responsible for pumping blood throughout all the body except the lungs. Consequently, its walls are three times thicker than those of the right ventricle and pressures in this chamber are up to six times greater.

There are well-developed trabeculae carneae and two large papillary muscles.

The region of the ventricle below the aorta is the aortic vestibule.

The mitral valve guards the left atrioventricular orifice. It is bicuspid (anterior and posterior), with attached chordae tendineae similar to the tricuspid valve.

The three-cusped aortic valve is similar to the pulmonary valve. Above each cusp the aortic wall bulges to form the aortic sinuses. The right aortic sinus gives rise to the right coronary artery; the left sinus gives origin to the left coronary artery.

The interventricular septum is of equal thickness to the left ventricle and consequently bulges into the right ventricle. Where it attaches to the fibrous ring, it is thinner and more fibrous—this is the membranous part of the septum.

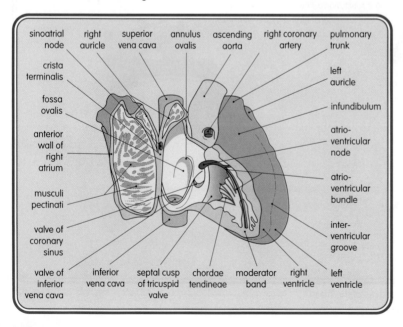

Fig. 3.17 Interior of right atrium and right ventricle.

Skeleton of the heart

The two atria and two ventricles are attached to a pair of fibrous rings around the atrioventricular orifice. The fibrous rings separate the muscle fibres of the atria and ventricles, with the atrioventricular conducting system forming the only physiological connection between the atria and ventricles.

The bases of the cusps of the atrioventricular valves and the membranous part of the atrioventricular septum are also attached to the fibrous skeleton.

Blood supply of the heart

Fig. 3.18 illustrates the blood supply of the heart.

Narrowing of the coronary arteries (ischaemic heart disease), usually due to atheromatous deposition in their walls, gives rise to conditions such as angina pectoris and myocardial infarction. Ischaemic heart disease is the commonest cause of death in the Western world. The anterior interventricular artery is most commonly affected.

Venous drainage of the heart

Most of the venous blood in the heart drains into the coronary sinus, which lies in the posterior atrioventricular groove. It is a continuation of the great cardiac vein, and opens into the right atrium.

The small and middle cardiac veins empty into the coronary sinus.

The remaining blood is returned to the heart via the anterior cardiac veins to the right atrium and other small veins (venae cordis minimae) that open directly into the heart chambers.

Conducting system of the heart

The heart contracts rhythmically at about 70 beats per minute.

The sinoatrial node (pacemaker) lies in the upper part of the sulcus terminalis. Impulses generated here are transmitted throughout the atria to the atrioventricular node, which lies in the atrial septum just above the attachment of the septal cusp of the tricuspid valve. The atrioventricular node conducts impulses to the bundle of His.

The bundle of His conducts the impulses to the inferior part of the interventricular septum. At this point the bundle divides into two branches, one for each ventricle:

- The right branch conducts the impulse to the apex of the right ventricle and, via the moderator band, to the anterior wall. The impulses are then distributed throughout the muscle.

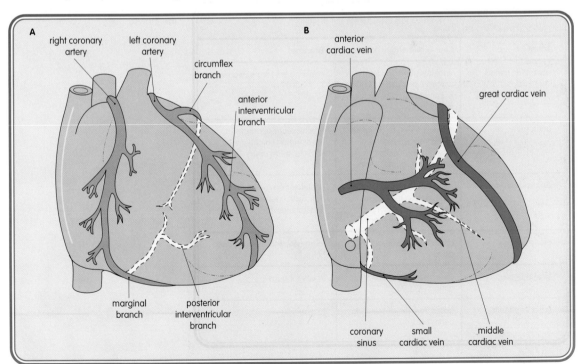

Fig. 3.18 Blood supply of the heart: (A) coronary arteries; (B) coronary veins.

- The left branch pierces the septum and passes down on the left side beneath the endocardium. It divides into two branches.

Fig. 3.19 details the nerve supply of the heart.

Great vessels of the thorax

Fig. 3.20 outlines the thoracic aorta and its branches.
Fig. 3.21 shows the aortic arch and pulmonary trunk.

Pulmonary trunk

This vessel transports deoxygenated blood from the right ventricle to the lungs.

The ligamentum arteriosum (see Fig. 3.21) is a fibrous band that connects the bifurcation of the pulmonary trunk to the aortic arch. It is the remnant of the ductus arteriosus, which in the foetus conducts blood from the pulmonary trunk to the aorta, bypassing the lungs.

Outline of the nerve supply of the heart		
Nerve type	**Origin**	**Action**
sympathetic nerves	cervical and upper thoracic part of the sympathetic trunk via the cardiac plexuses	increase the rate and force of contraction
parasympathetic nerves	vagus nerves via the cardiac plexuses	reduce the rate and force of contraction

Fig. 3.19 Outline of the nerve supply of the heart.

Aorta and its branches in the thorax		
Artery	**Course and origin**	**Branches**
ascending aorta	originates from the left ventricle, and ascends and becomes the aortic arch at the sternal angle	right and left coronary arteries
aortic arch	arches posteriorly to the left of the trachea and the oesophagus, and continues as the descending aorta	brachiocephalic artery, left common carotid artery, left subclavian artery
descending aorta	descends to the left of the vertebral column and leaves the thorax by passing through the diaphragm	posterior intercostal arteries, subcostal arteries and visceral branches
bronchial	arises from the descending aorta	to bronchi and visceral pleura
oesophageal	arises from the descending aorta	to oesophagus
superior phrenic	arises from the descending aorta	to diaphragm

Fig. 3.20 Aorta and its branches in the thorax.

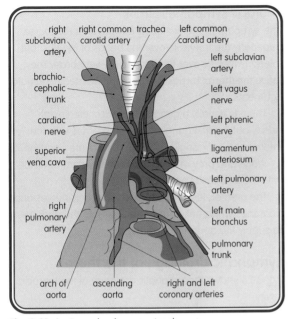

Fig. 3.21 Aorta and pulmonary trunk.

Superior vena cava

The superior vena cava drains the upper limbs and the head and neck. It drains into the right atrium and receives the azygos vein before it enters the pericardium.

Inferior vena cava

The vein pierces the central tendon of the diaphragm opposite T8 vertebra and almost immediately enters the right atrium.

Fig. 3.22 shows the superior and inferior venae cavae and their main tributaries.

Pulmonary veins

Two pulmonary veins leave each lung, carrying oxygenated blood to the left atrium of the heart.

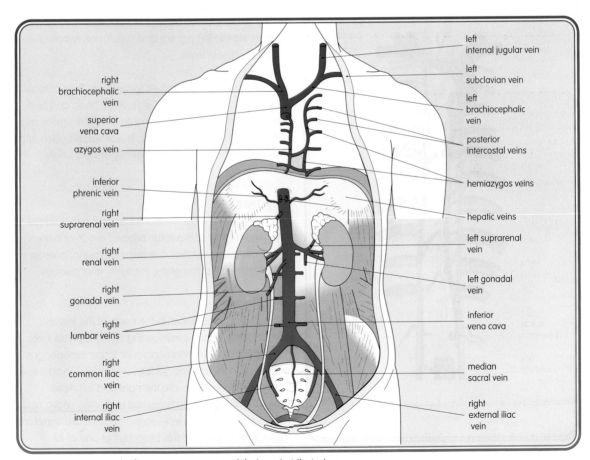

Fig. 3.22 Superior and inferior venae cavae and their main tributaries.

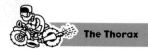

Azygos system of veins

Fig. 3.23 shows the azygos system of veins and the thoracic duct.

Nerves of the thorax

Fig. 3.24 lists the main nerves of the thorax (see also Fig. 3.15).

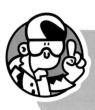

The vagus passes behind the root of the lung; the phrenic nerve passes in front of the lung root.

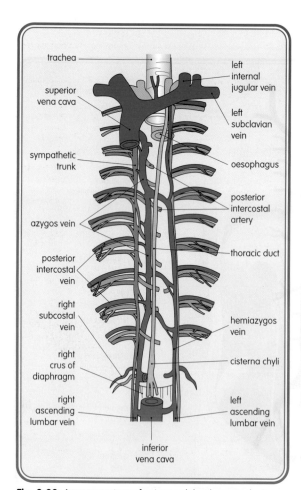

Fig. 3.23 Azygos system of veins and the thoracic duct.

Thoracic sympathetic trunk

The sympathetic trunks follow a paravertebral course. Superiorly the trunks lie over the heads of the ribs, but inferiorly they lie over the body of the vertebrae. They leave the thorax by passing through the medial arcuate ligaments.

There is usually a ganglion for each intercostal nerve, but the first ganglion usually merges with the inferior cervical ganglion to form the stellate ganglion.

White and grey rami communicantes communicate with the intercostal nerves.

The greater, lesser, and least splanchnic nerves arise from the sympathetic trunk and pass into the abdomen to supply the abdominal contents.

Lymphatic drainage of the thorax

Fig. 3.25 shows the lymphatic drainage of the thoracic cavity.

The thoracic duct (see Fig. 3.23) receives lymph from:
- The lower half of the body.
- The left posterior intercostal nodes.
- The left side of the head and neck, and the left upper limb, via the left jugular and subclavian lymph trunks, respectively.

The right lymph duct receives lymph from the posterior right thoracic wall. The right side of the head and neck, and the right upper limb drain into the right jugular and subclavian trunks, respectively. These vessels open into the great veins either independently or as a single trunk, the right lymph trunk.

Thymus

This is the major organ responsible for the maturation of T lymphocytes. It is a large bilobed organ at birth, lying in the superior and anterior mediastina, anterior to the great vessels. The gland involutes after puberty.

Trachea

The trachea commences in the neck, at the lower border of the cricoid cartilage (Fig. 3.26). It passes into the superior mediastinum, anterior to the oesophagus and close to the midline. At the level of T4–T5 vertebrae, the trachea bifurcates into the right and left main bronchi. The right main bronchus is shorter, wider, and more vertical than the left—foreign bodies are therefore more likely to lodge in this bronchus or one of its branches.

Nerves of the thorax	
Nerve (origin)	**Course and distribution**
vagus (X and medulla oblongata)	enters superior mediastinum posterior to sternoclavicular joint and brachiocephalic vein to supply pulmonary plexus, oesophageal plexus, and cardiac plexus
phrenic (anterior rami of C3–C5)	enters thorax and runs between mediastinal pleura and pericardium to supply motor and sensory innervation to diaphragm
intercostals (anterior rami of T1–T11)	runs between internal and innermost layers of intercostal muscles and supplies skin and muscles of each intercostal space
subcostal (anterior ramus of T12)	follows inferior border of 12th rib and passes into abdominal wall
recurrent laryngeal (X)	loops around subclavian on right and arch of aorta on left, and ascends in tracheoesophageal groove; supplies intrinsic muscles of larynx (except cricothyroid) and sensation inferior to level of vocal folds
cardiac plexus (X and sympathetic trunks)	fibres pass along coronary arteries to sinoatrial node; parasympathetic fibres reduce heart rate and force of contraction, sympathetic fibres increase rate and contraction force
pulmonary plexus (X and sympathetic trunks)	plexus forms on root of lung and extends along branches of bronchi; parasympathetic fibres constrict bronchioles, sympathetic fibres dilate them
oesophageal (X sympathetic ganglia and greater splanchnic nerve)	vagus and sympathetic nerves form a plexus around oesophagus to supply smooth muscle and glands of inferior two-thirds of oesophagus

Fig. 3.24 Nerves of the thorax.

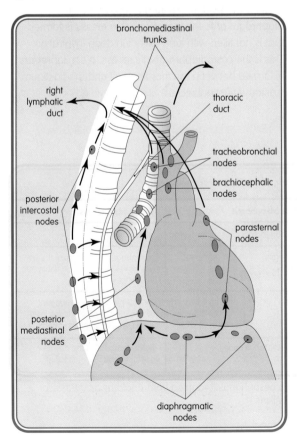

Fig. 3.25 Lymphatic drainage of the thoracic cavity.

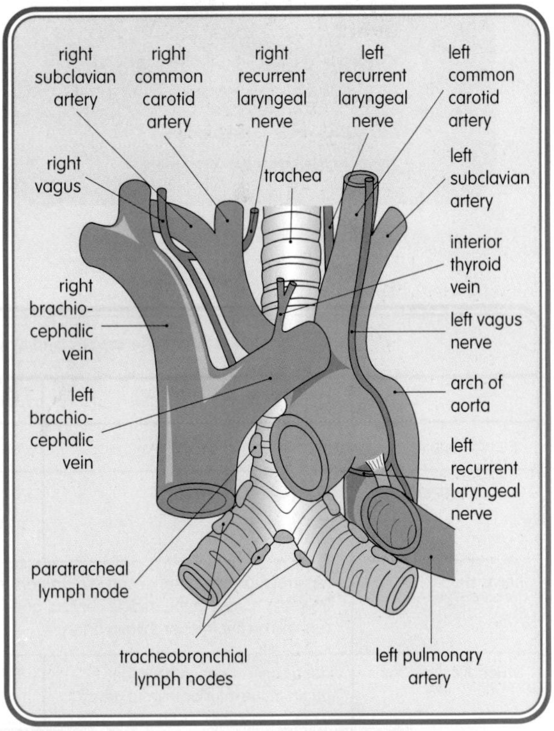

Fig. 3.26 Trachea and its main relations anteriorly and laterally.

Oesophagus

This organ commences as a continuation of the laryngopharynx at the level of C6 vertebra. In the thorax the oesophagus lies between the trachea and the vertebral column. It then passes through the diaphragm at the level of T10 vertebra and after 1–2 cm enters the stomach. Fibres from the right crus of the diaphragm form a sling around the oesophagus.

The upper oesophageal sphincter lies at the level of cricopharyngeus. This is the narrowest part of the oesophagus. Other constrictions in the oesophagus are found where it is crossed by the aortic arch and left main bronchus, and where it pierces the diaphragm.

Fig. 3.27 outlines the blood supply, lymphatic drainage, and nerve supply of the oesophagus.

- List the divisions of the mediastinum and their contents.
- Define the structure and blood supply of the heart.
- Outline the great vessels of the thorax.
- Discuss the lymphatic drainage of the thorax.

PLEURAE AND LUNGS

Pleurae

The pleurae surround the lungs. The pleura is divided into two layers, the parietal and visceral pleurae (Fig. 3.28).

The parietal pleura lines the thoracic wall (costal pleura), the thoracic surface of the diaphragm (diaphragmatic pleura), and the lateral aspect of the mediastinum (mediastinal pleura). At the thoracic inlet it arches over the lungs as the cervical pleura. It lies above the clavicle at this point.

The visceral pleura completely invests the outer surface of the lung and invaginates into the fissures of the lungs. Consequently, it is firmly adherent to the lungs.

The two layers become continuous with each other at the root of the lung. Here there is a double layer of pleura that hangs down as the pulmonary ligament.

The pleural cavity lies between the two pleural layers. It is a potential space and, in health, contains a small quantity of clear pleural fluid.

Where the parietal pleura is reflected off the diaphragm onto the thoracic wall, a recess is formed that is not filled with lung except in deep inspiration. This is the costodiaphragmatic recess. A similar recess is formed between the thoracic wall and mediastinum (costomediastinal recess).

Blood and nerve supply, and lymphatic drainage of the oesophagus			
	Upper oesophagus	**Middle oesophagus**	**Lower oesophagus**
arterial supply	inferior thyroid artery	oesophageal branches of the aorta	left gastric artery
venous drainage	brachiocephalic vein	azygos vein	oesophageal tributaries of the left gastric veins which drain finally into the portal vein
nerve supply	recurrent laryngeal nerve and sympathetic fibres from cell bodies in the middle cervical ganglion running on the inferior thyroid artery		fibres from the anterior and posterior oesophageal plexus from the vagus nerve; sympathetic fibres from the sympathetic trunk and greater splanchnic nerve
lymphatic drainage	deep cervical nodes near the origin of the inferior thyroid artery	tracheobronchial nodes	preaortic nodes of the coeliac group

Fig. 3.27 Blood and nerve supply, and lymphatic drainage of the oesophagus. (Adapted from *Anatomy as a Basis for Clinical Medicine*, by E.C.B. Hall-Craggs. Courtesy of Williams & Wilkins.)

The nerve supply of the parietal pleura is described in Fig. 3.29. The visceral pleura has no somatic innervation and is therefore insensitive to pain.

Blood supply of the pleurae

The parietal pleura is supplied by the intercostal arteries and branches of the internal thoracic artery. Venous drainage and lymphatic drainage are similarly shared.

The visceral pleura is supplied by the bronchial arteries. It shares venous and lymphatic drainage with the lung.

Endothoracic fascia

This layer of loose connective tissue separates the parietal pleura from the thoracic wall. It includes the suprapleural membrane, which covers the dome of the parietal pleura where it projects into the root of the neck.

Lungs

The lungs in life are light, spongy, and elastic. The surface changes from a pink colour at birth to a mottled darker colour in later life because of deposition of carbon particles from atmospheric pollution. This is more pronounced in city-dwellers and smokers.

Each lung lies free in the pleural cavity except at its root, where it is attached to the mediastinum.

Surfaces and borders of the lungs

These are indicated in Figs 3.30 and 3.31. Each lung has an apex that projects into the neck about 1 cm above the clavicle, a base that lies against the diaphragm, a costal surface, and a mediastinal surface.

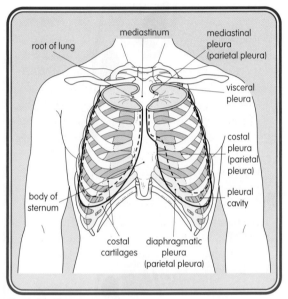

Fig. 3.28 Pleurae.

Nerve supply of the parietal pleura	
Pleura	**Nerve supply**
costal	segmentally by the intercostal nerves
mediastinal	the phrenic nerve
diaphragmatic	the phrenic nerve centrally, the lower five intercostal nerves peripherally
visceral	autonomic nerve supply from the pulmonary plexus

Fig. 3.29 Nerve supply of the parietal pleura.

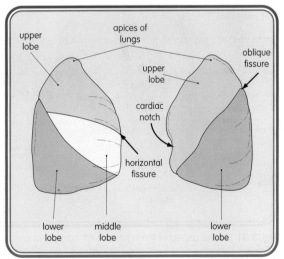

Fig. 3.30 Surface of the lungs.

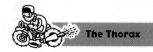

The hilum (root) of the lung (see Fig. 3.31) lies on the mediastinal surface where the bronchi and neurovascular bundles enter the lungs.

Bronchi and bronchopulmonary segments

The trachea divides into the right and left main bronchi. These are fibromuscular tubes reinforced by incomplete

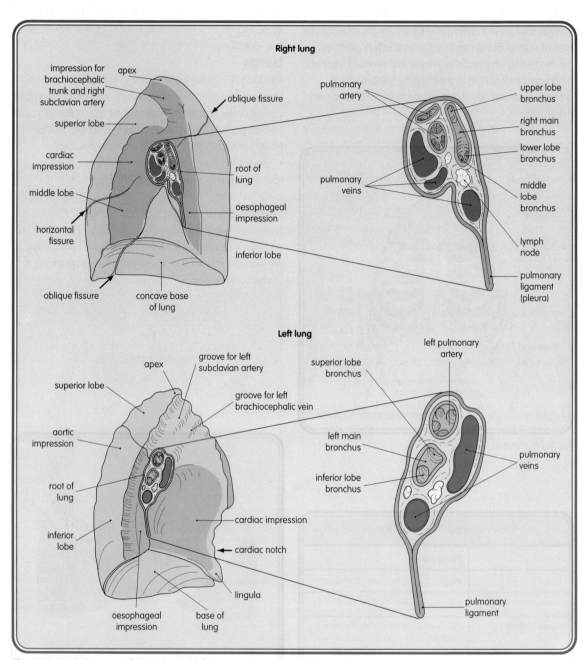

Fig. 3.31 Medial aspect of the right and left lungs and contents of their roots.

rings of cartilage. They are lined by respiratory epithelium.

In the lung, the main bronchus divides into secondary (lobar) bronchi, which in turn divide into tertiary (segmental) bronchi. The latter supply the bronchopulmonary segments, the functional units of the lungs.

Bronchopulmonary segments are wedge shaped, with the base lying peripherally and the apex lying towards the root of the lungs. There are 10 segments for each lung. Each segment has its own segmental bronchus, segmental artery, lymphatic vessels, and autonomic nerves. The veins lie both in and between segments. Within each segment the segmental bronchus repeatedly subdivides and reduces in size until the cartilage in the walls disappears. The airway is now called a bronchiole. These subdivide and eventually give rise to the alveoli, which are thin-walled sacs with no muscle in the wall. These subdivisions greatly increase the surface area of the lungs, allowing efficient exchange of gases.

Nerve supply of the lungs
Sympathetic and parasympathetic nerves from the pulmonary plexuses, which lie anterior and posterior to the lung roots, supply the smooth muscle of the bronchial tree, the vessels, and the mucous membrane.

Blood supply of the lungs
The lungs have a dual blood supply:
- Bronchial arteries from the thoracic aorta supply the bronchi, the connective tissue of the lung, and the visceral pleura. Bronchial veins drain into the azygos system of veins.
- Pulmonary arteries transport deoxygenated blood to the alveolar capillaries. The pulmonary veins return oxygenated blood to the lungs.

There are anastomoses between the pulmonary and bronchial circulations.

Pulmonary thromboembolism is a common cause of morbidity and mortality in the UK. Approximately 10% of hospital patients develop a pulmonary embolus; although most cases are silent, in severe cases this can lead to pulmonary infarction or sudden death. The source of the embolus is often from the deep veins of the legs.

Lymphatic drainage of the lungs
Fig. 3.32 illustrates the lymphatic drainage of the lungs.

Bronchial carcinoma is the most common lethal cancer in the UK and USA. It usually spreads via the lymphatics, and has a poor prognosis. An understanding of the anatomy and lymphatic drainage is essential for planning treatment and assessing the prognosis of these tumours.

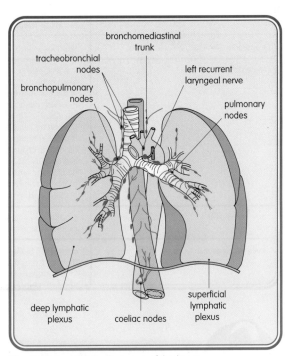

Fig. 3.32 Lymphatic drainage of the lungs.

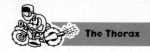

Mechanics of respiration

Respiration consists of an inspiratory and an expiratory phase (Fig. 3.33).

Patients with severe obstruction of the airways, e.g. severe asthma or chronic obstructive airways disease, can be seen using their accessory muscles of respiration, which include the sternocleido mastoids, pectoralis, scalene, and anterior abdominal muscles. Signs include intercostal recession, suprasternal recession, pursing of the lips, and contraction of the sternomastoid and platysma.

Fig. 3.33 Movements and muscles involved in respiration.

Movements and muscles involved in respiration	
Movement	**Muscles involved**
quiet inspiration	
increased vertical diameter	contraction of the diaphragm, causing flattening of the domes; this is the major muscle of quiet inspiration
increased anteroposterior diameter	elevation of the ribs at their sternal ends, pushing the sternum forwards; this is achieved by contraction of the scalenus muscles, to fix the 1st rib, and contraction of the intercostal muscles, which raises all of the ribs towards the 1st rib
transverse diameter	elevation of the ribs as described above
forced inspiration	the scalene muscles and sternomastoid elevate the ribs, producing some movement at themanubriosternal joint; the intercostal muscles contract more forcefully, elevating the ribs; the 12th rib is fixed by quadratus lumbarum, allowing a more forceful downward movement of the diaphragm: as inspiration further increases, the back is arched by the erector spinae muscles, and the pectoral girdle is stabilized by grasping a heavy object, allowing the pectoral muscles to help elevate the ribs
quiet expiration	passive movement brought about by the elastic recoil of the lungs
forced expiration	contraction of the anterior abdominal wall muscles forces the diaphragm upwards and depresses the ribs

- Describe the pleura.
- Outline the anatomy of the lung.
- Discuss the mechanics of respiration.

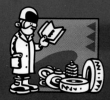

4. The Abdomen

REGIONS AND COMPONENTS OF THE ABDOMEN

The abdominal cavity is separated from the thoracic cavity by the diaphragm. Because the domes of the diaphragm arch high above the costal margin, the upper part of the abdomen—including the liver, the spleen, the upper poles of the kidneys, and the suprarenal glands—is protected by the bony thoracic cage. The lower part of the abdominal cavity lies in the bony pelvis.

Posteriorly, the vertebral column protects the abdominal contents, but anteriorly and laterally the abdomen is more vulnerable to injury, with only a muscular wall for protection.

The anterolateral abdominal wall is made up of a muscular sheet composed of three muscle layers.

These are separated laterally but fuse anteriorly to surround the rectus abdominis.

The abdominal cavity contains most of the alimentary tract (stomach, duodenum, and small and large intestines) together with its derivatives (liver, spleen, and pancreas). Parts of the viscera (e.g. small intestines and transverse colon) are attached to double folds of peritoneum, called mesentery, whilst others (e.g. duodenum) are bound down to the posterior abdominal wall. The kidney, suprarenal glands, and ureters lie in the posterior abdominal wall, behind the peritoneum.

Abdominal pain is a very common presentation— knowledge of the embryology and anatomy of the region is crucial in obtaining the correct diagnosis (Fig. 4.1).

Origin and blood supply of the abdominal viscera			
Part of fetal gut	Organs	Blood supply	Usual site of presentation of abdominal pain
foregut	oesophagus, stomach, first part of duodenum, liver, spleen, pancreas	coeliac artery	epigastric region
midgut	remainder of duodenum, jejunum, ileum, caecum, appendix, ascending colon, right two-thirds of transverse colon	superior mesenteric artery	umbilical region
hindgut	remainder of transverse colon, descending colon, rectum	inferior mesenteric artery	suprapubic region

Fig. 4.1 Origin and blood supply of the abdominal viscera.

SURFACE ANATOMY AND SUPERFICIAL STRUCTURES

To facilitate description, the abdomen is divided into regions. The simplest method is to divide the abdomen into four quadrants by vertical and horizontal lines through the umbilicus; however, for more accurate description, it is divided into nine regions by two vertical and two horizontal lines (Fig. 4.2):

- The vertical line on each side corresponds to the midclavicular line, which extends down to the midinguinal point.
- The lower transverse line runs between the two tubercles of the iliac crest (intertubercular plane).
- The upper transverse line lies midway between the pubic symphysis and jugular notch (transpyloric plane).

The linea alba is a midline depression running from the xiphisternum to the umbilicus. The linea semilunaris is a smooth, curved line, representing the lateral margin of the rectus abdominis. The fundus of the gall bladder lies deep to where the linea semilunaris intersects the costal margin.

The inguinal ligament runs from the anterior superior iliac spine to the pubic tubercle. The deep inguinal ring lies at the midinguinal point (halfway between the anterior superior iliac spine and the pubic tubercle).

○ **Outline the surface anatomy of the abdomen.**

THE ABDOMINAL WALL

Skeleton

Fig. 4.3 shows the skeleton of the abdominal and pelvic cavities.

The costal margin and floating ribs have been described previously (see Chapter 3).

The hip bones articulate with the sacrum at the sacroiliac joint and with each other at the pubic symphysis. Each pelvic bone is formed by an iliac bone, ischium, and pubic bone.

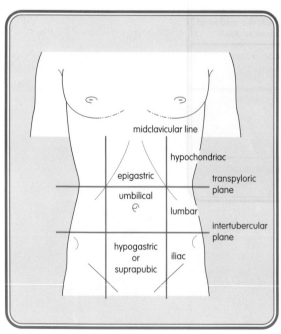

Fig. 4.2 Regions of the abdomen.

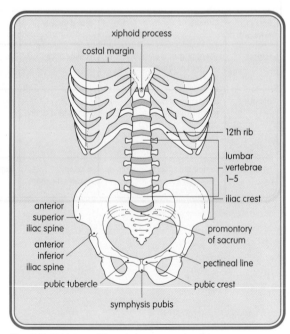

Fig. 4.3 Skeleton of the abdomen and pelvis.

The iliac bones protect the underlying structures, providing a site for muscle attachment. The upper border, the iliac crest, is limited by the anterior superior iliac spine (ASIS) and the posterior superior iliac spine (PSIS), anteriorly and posteriorly, respectively. The iliac tubercle lies behind the ASIS.

The three sheets of muscle of the anterolateral abdominal wall arise from the iliac crest. The latissimus dorsi, quadratus lumborum, and thoracolumbar fascia are also attached to the crest.

The pectineal line represents the area of fusion between the ileum and the superior ramus of the pubic bone. Medial to this line lie the pubic tubercle and pubic crest.

Thoracolumbar fascia

This arises from:
- Tips of the lumbar spines.
- Tips of the lumbar transverse processes.
- The anterior aspect of the lumbar transverse processes.

The anterior and middle sheets enclose the quadratus lumborum muscle; the middle and posterior sheets enclose the erector spinae muscle. The three sheets fuse laterally and provide attachment for the internal oblique and transverse abdominis muscles.

Muscles of the anterolateral abdominal wall

Fig. 4.4 outlines the muscles of the anterolateral abdominal wall.

Rectus sheath

Each rectus abdominis muscle is enclosed in a fibrous sheath formed by the aponeurotic tendons of the three lateral muscles (Fig. 4.5).

The external oblique muscle contributes to the anterior layer of the sheath over its entire extent. Below the costal margin, the internal oblique aponeurosis splits around the muscle, forming the anterior and posterior layers. The aponeurosis of transversus abdominis contributes to the posterior layer.

Midway between the symphysis pubis and the umbilicus, the posterior wall of the sheath becomes deficient, and all the aponeuroses pass anterior to the rectus muscle. The free posterior margin thus formed is

Muscles of the anterolateral abdominal wall			
Name of muscle (nerve supply)	**Origin**	**Insertion**	**Action**
external oblique (T6–T12 spinal nerves, iliohypogastric and ilioinguinal nerves)	lower ribs	becomes aponeurotic and attaches to the xiphoid process, linea alba, pubic crest, pubic tubercle, and iliac crest	flexes and rotates trunk; pulls down ribs in forced expiration
internal oblique (spinal nerves T6–T12, iliohypogastric and ilioinguinal nerves)	lumbar fascia, iliac crest, lateral two-thirds of inguinal ligament	lower three ribs and costal cartilages, xiphoid process, linea alba, symphysis pubis; forms conjoint tendon with transversus	assists in flexing and rotating trunk; pulls down ribs in forced expiration
transversus abdominis (spinal nerves T6–T12, iliohypogastric and ilioinguinal nerves)	lower six costal cartilages, lumbar fascia, iliac crest, lateral third of inguinal ligament	xiphoid process, linea alba, symphysis pubis	compresses abdominal contents with external and internal oblique
rectus abdominis (spinal nerves T6–T12)	symphysis pubis and pubic crest	costal cartilages 5–7 and xiphoid process	compresses abdominal contents and flexes vertebral column

Fig. 4.4 Muscles of the anterolateral abdominal wall.

called the the arcuate line. The inferior epigastric artery enters the sheath here and runs on the deep surface of rectus abdominis.

The posterior wall of the sheath is also deficient above the costal margin, where the rectus muscle lies directly on the underlying costal cartilages.

The body wall has three muscle layers in the abdomen. These layers fuse centrally to form the rectus sheath.

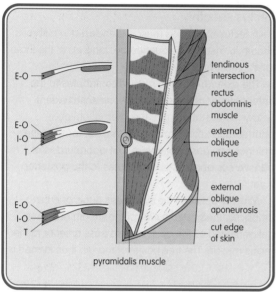

Fig. 4.5 Rectus sheath and rectus abdominis muscle. (E-O, external oblique; I-O, internal oblique; T, tendon.)

Nerve and blood supply to the anterolateral abdominal wall

The principal nerves and arteries of the anterolateral abdominal wall are shown in Fig. 4.6.

Venous drainage of the anterolateral abdominal wall

The superficial veins include the superficial epigastric and thoracoepigastric veins. These drain ultimately into the femoral vein and axillary veins, respectively.

The superior and inferior epigastric veins and the deep circumflex iliac veins follow the arteries and drain into the internal thoracic and external iliac veins.

The lower two posterior intercostal veins drain into the azygos veins. The lumbar veins drain into the inferior vena cava. Blood may return to the heart via the

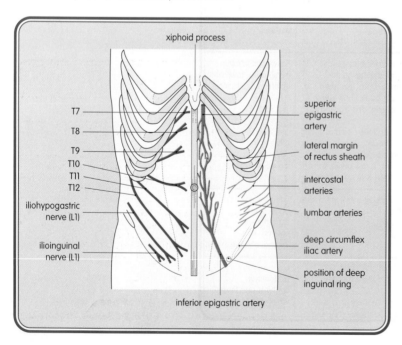

Fig. 4.6 Innervation (left) and arterial supply (right) of the anterolateral abdominal wall.

superficial abdominal veins if the inferior vena cava becomes obstructed.

Inguinal region

Inguinal ligament

This is the lower free edge of the aponeurosis of the external oblique muscle. It extends from the ASIS to the pubic tubercle and gives origin to the internal oblique and transverse abdominis muscles and the fascia lata of the thigh.

Inguinal canal

This is an oblique narrow slit, about 6 cm long, lying above the medial half of the inguinal ligament (Figs 4.7 and 4.8). It commences at the deep inguinal ring and ends at the superficial ring. The canal contains the spermatic cord and the ilioinguinal nerve in males, and the round ligament and the ilioinguinal nerve in females.

The superficial inguinal ring is a triangular slit in the external oblique aponeurosis, just above and lateral to the pubic tubercle. The contents of the inguinal canal exit through this ring.

The deep inguinal ring lies at the midinguinal point and is an opening in the transversalis fascia. The contents of the spermatic cord pass through the deep inguinal ring.

The ilioinguinal nerve does not enter the inguinal canal through the inguinal ring but via the anterior wall of the canal, by running between the external oblique aponeurosis and the internal oblique muscle.

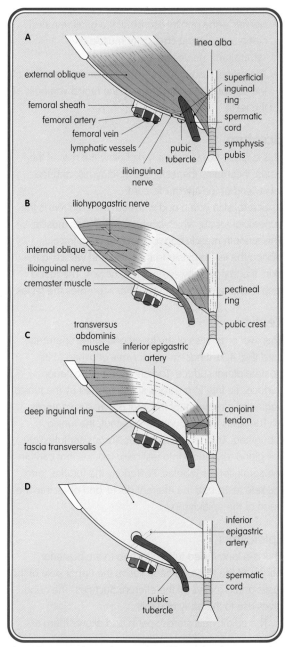

Fig. 4.7 Inguinal canal viewed at different levels. (A) Superficial inguinal ring in external oblique muscle. (B, C) Internal oblique and transversus muscles and the conjoint tendon. (C) Deep inguinal ring in fascia transversalis.

Composition of the inguinal canal	
Region	**Components**
anterior wall	external oblique aponeurosis; reinforced laterally by internal oblique
floor	lower edge of the inguinal ligament; reinforced medially by the lacunar ligament, which lies between the inguinal ligament and the pectineal line
roof	lower edges of the internal oblique and transversus muscles: these muscles arch over the front of the cord laterally, to behind the cord medially, where their joint tendon—the conjoint tendon—is inserted into the pubic crest and pectineal line of the pubic bone
posterior wall	the strong conjoint tendon medially and the weak transversalis fascia laterally

Fig. 4.8 Composition of the inguinal canal.

Spermatic cord

The structures entering the deep inguinal ring pick up three coverings from the layers of the abdominal wall as they pass through the canal to form the spermatic cord (Fig. 4.9). The spermatic cord with all of its coverings is not complete until it emerges from the superficial inguinal ring.

Contents of the spermatic cord comprise: (10 가장)
- The ductus deferens.

- Arteries—the testicular artery (from the abdominal aorta) and the artery to the ductus deferens (from the superior and inferior vesical arteries).
- Veins—the pampiniform plexus of veins.
- Lymphatics—accompany the veins from the testis to the para-aortic nodes.
- Nerves—the genital branch of the genitofemoral nerve supplies the cremaster muscle and sympathetic nerves go to the arteries.
- The processus vaginalis—the obliterated remains of the peritoneal connection with the tunica vaginalis of the testis.

Scrotum

This is a sac-like structure lying below the root of the penis. It contains the testis, the epididymis, and the lower end of the spermatic cord.

Scrotal skin is thin and wrinkled. Beneath this is the superficial fascia, which contains the dartos muscle. This smooth muscle contracts in response to cold, pulling the testes closer to the body and wrinkling the skin. It is supplied by sympathetic nerves. The fascia also forms a median partition that separates the testes.

Testis

This oval organ lies at the lower end of the spermatic cord (Fig. 4.9). It has the epididymis attached to its posterolateral surface. The anterior and posterior surfaces lie free in a serous space formed by the tunica vaginalis, a remnant of the fetal processus vaginalis.

The testis has a tough fibrous coat, the tunica albuginea. This sends numerous fibrous septules into the gland, dividing it into testicular lobules that contain the seminiferous tubules. Posteriorly the tubules form the rete testis and the efferent ducts, and open into the head of the epididymis.

Epididymis

This is a long coiled tube attached to the posterior border of the testis. Its head lies at the upper pole of the testis and is joined by the efferent ductules. The head gives rise to the body and tail.

The epididymis stores sperm and allows them to mature.

Ductus deferens

This tube transmits sperm from the testis and epididymis to the prostatic urethra.

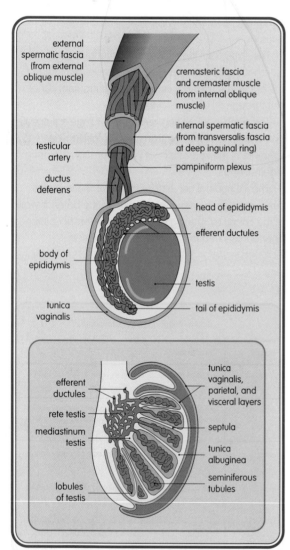

Fig. 4.9 Left testis, epididymis, coverings, and contents of the spermatic cord.

Blood supply of the testis

The testicular artery runs in the spermatic cord and supplies the testis and the epididymis. The pampiniform plexus provides venous drainage. In the inguinal canal the plexus merges into four veins, which join to form two veins that leave the deep inguinal ring. The left testicular vein drains into the left renal vein, and the right into the inferior vena cava. Renal tumours may obstruct the left renal vein, causing dilatation of the veins in the testis, to form a varicocoele.

The testicular artery and its branches are very closely associated with the pampiniform venous plexus. This acts as a countercurrent heat exchanger. For spermatogenesis to occur, the testicular temperature has to be 2–3°C below body temperature.

Lymphatics drain into the para-aortic nodes.

Descent of the testis

The testis develops in the posterior abdominal wall of the embryo, but then migrates—through the inguinal canal—into the scrotum: it reaches the deep inguinal ring by 4 months and inside the canal at 7 months, then progresses rapidly through the superficial ring to reach the scrotum at around the time of birth.

A diverticulum of peritoneum, the processus vaginalis, precedes the testis as it passes through the inguinal canal into the scrotum. The processus is normally obliterated except at its lower end, where it becomes the tunica vaginalis.

The mechanism of descent of the testis is not known but it is preceded by a gubernaculum. This does not pull the testis down.

The cremaster muscle elevates the testes towards the inguinal canal as part of the cremasteric reflex. This reflex is very active in children, often leading to a misdiagnosis of undescended testes. Failure of the testis to descend is a serious condition—it may result in impaired fertility, and undescended testes may undergo malignant change.

A hernia is a protrusion of a viscus or part of a viscus through its coverings into an abnormal situation, most frequently into the inguinal canal (inguinal hernia). Direct hernias are common in adults and result from a defect in the mucle layers of the abdominal wall. The hernia pushes through the posterior wall of the inguinal canal and its neck lies medial to the inferior epigastric artery. Indirect hernias are seen often in babies and result from failure of the processus vaginalis to

obliterate. There is no defect in the abdominal wall and the hernia passes through the inguinal canal and may enter the scrotum.

- Describe the skeleton and muscles of the abdominal wall.
- What is the rectus sheath?
- Outline the anatomy of the inguinal canal.
- List the contents of the spermatic cord.
- Outline the anatomy of the testis, epididymis, and scrotum.

THE PERITONEUM

This is a serous membrane lined by mesothelium. It has two layers continuous with each other :

- The parietal layer covers the anterior and posterior abdominal wall, the inferior surface of the diaphragm, and the pelvic cavity.
- The visceral layer leaves the abdominal wall and invests the viscera to a greater or lesser degree. This is the serous covering for many of the viscera.

Embryology

During development, the foregut, midgut, and hindgut are suspended from the posterior abdominal wall by a dorsal mesentery (a mesentery is a double layer of peritoneum that encloses an organ and connects it to the body wall—Fig. 4.10). These organs are intraperitoneal.

Some organs lie against the posterior abdominal wall and are covered by peritoneum on their anterior surface only (e.g. the kidneys). These organs are retroperitoneal.

A ventral mesentery is present only in the terminal parts of the oesophagus and stomach, and the upper part of the duodenum (foregut). It is derived from the septum transversum. Growth of the liver divides the mesentery into the falciform ligament and the lesser omentum.

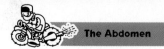

Nerve supply of the peritoneum

The parietal peritoneum is supplied segmentally by the nerves supplying the overlying muscles and skin. The peritoneum covering the inferior surface of the diaphragm is supplied by the intercostal nerves peripherally and by the phrenic nerve centrally. The visceral peritoneum does not have a somatic innervation and is therefore insensitive to pain.

The diaphragm and its innervation originate in the neck. Irritation of the diaphragm by abdominal or thoracic pathology may cause pain in the shoulder tips. This is termed 'referred pain'.

Peritoneal folds of the anterolateral abdominal wall

These are shown in Fig. 4.11 and include:
- Median umbilical fold—contains the remnant of urachus (median umbilical ligaments).
- Medial umbilical fold—contains remnants of the umbilical arteries (medial umbilical ligaments).
- Lateral umbilical fold—contains the inferior epigastric vessels.

The falciform ligament contains the ligamentum teres (the remnant of the umbilical vein) in its free margin.

Greater and lesser sacs

The space between the parietal and visceral peritoneum is only potential and contains a small quantity of peritoneal fluid. This is the greater sac or general peritoneal cavity.

The lesser sac (omental bursa) is a diverticulum of the peritoneal cavity behind the stomach. It forms because of the change in position of the liver, stomach, and spleen during development. The lesser sac communicates with the greater sac through the epiploic foramen.

Greater and lesser omenta

The greater omentum arises from the greater curvature of the stomach and the superior duodenum. It is filled with fat. The transverse colon and its mesentery are fused to the posterior aspect of the omentum.

The lesser omentum connects the lesser curvature of the stomach and the proximal part of the duodenum to the liver.

Fig. 4.10 The embryonic dorsal (A) and ventral (B) mesenteries and the formation of the retroperitoneal part of the intestines (C and D). (Adapted from *Anatomy as a Basis for Clinical Medicine*, by E.C.B. Hall-Craggs. Courtesy of Williams & Wilkins.)

The greater omentum is the 'policeman' of the abdomen—it can be passively moved to a site of infection and adhere to it, preventing spread.

⊙ **Describe the peritoneum of the abdomen.**

THE ABDOMINAL ORGANS

Oesophagus

After passing through the diaphragm, the oesophagus turns forward and to the left to enter the cardiac part of the stomach. Blood and nerve supply are shown in Fig. 3.26.

Gastro-oesophageal reflux is a very common problem in young children and in adults. A number of factors normally prevent reflux of stomach contents into the oesophagus. These include:

- The sphincteric action of the lower oesophageal muscle.
- The sling of the right crus making an angle between the oesophagus and stomach.
- A mucosal flap.
- Positive intra-abdominal pressure and negative intrathoracic pressure.

Stomach

This is a dilated muscular bag lying between the oesophagus and the duodenum (Fig. 4.12). It is a relatively mobile organ, being fixed at its ends. The gastro-oesophageal junction lies at the level of T10 vertebra, and the pyloric sphincter (gastroduodenal sphincter) lies at the level of L1 vertebra.

The stomach is capable of considerable dilation and thus has a rugose inner surface. The mucosa is extensively folded, and there is an outer longitudinal, middle circular, and inner incomplete oblique muscle layer.

The relations of the stomach comprise:

- Anterior—the anterolateral abdominal wall, left costal margin, and diaphragm.
- Posterior (stomach bed)—the left suprarenal gland, upper pole of the left kidney, pancreas, spleen, and left colic flexure.

The stomach and oesphagus are foregut derivatives and therefore get their blood supply from the coeliac trunk, a branch of the abdominal aorta (see Fig. 4.12).

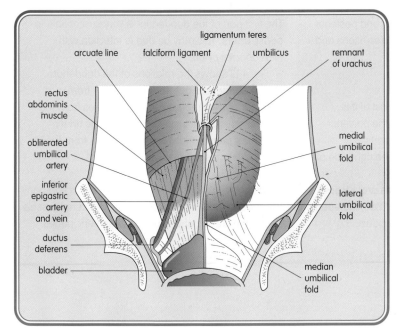

Fig. 4.11 Peritoneal folds of the anterior abdominal wall.

ligamentum teres
arcuate line
falciform ligament
umbilicus
remnant of urachus
rectus abdominis muscle
obliterated umbilical artery
medial umbilical fold
inferior epigastric artery and vein
lateral umbilical fold
ductus deferens
bladder
median umbilical fold

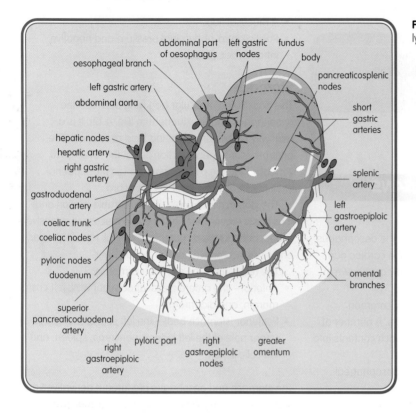

Fig. 4.12 Blood supply and lymphatic drainage of the stomach.

Lymphatic drainage is illustrated in Fig. 4.12.

The nerve supply to the stomach and oesophagus comprises:

- Sympathetic—from the coeliac plexus distributed along arteries.
- Parasympathetic—from the anterior and posterior vagal trunks. Stimulation increases secretions and peristaltic activity.

Duodenum

The duodenum is a C-shaped tube. Most of it is retroperitoneal and firmly attached to the posterior abdominal wall. It is divided into four parts:

- The first part passes posteriorly to the right side of the vertebral column.
- The second part passes downwards and receives the hepatopancreatic ampulla (of Vater), the opening of the bile duct and main pancreatic duct.
- The third part crosses the vertebral column at the level of L3 vertebra.
- The fourth part ascends to the level of L2 vertebra and opens into the jejunum.

The first part of the duodenum is very susceptible to peptic ulcers. This may be due to infection with *Helicobacter pylori*.

Fig. 4.13 shows the relations of the duodenum. The duodenum gets its blood supply from:

- Superior pancreaticoduodenal arteries from the gastroduodenal branch of the hepatic artery.
- Inferior pancreaticoduodenal arteries from the superior mesenteric artery.

Duodenal lymph drains into channels that accompany the superior and inferior pancreaticoduodenal vessels and to the coeliac and superior mesenteric nodes.

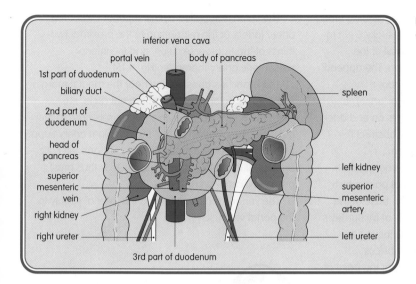

Fig. 4.13 Relations of the duodenum.

Jejunum and ileum

The jejunum and ileum lie free in the abdomen. They are attached to the posterior abdominal wall by the mesentery. Their total length is approximately 6–7 metres.

Fig. 4.14 outlines the differences between the jejunum and ileum.

Distinguishing characteristics of the jejunum and ileum		
Characteristic	Jejunum	Ileum
colour	deeper red	paler pink
wall	thick and heavy	thin and light
vascularity	greater	less
vasa recta	long	short
arcades	a few large loops	many short loops
fat in mesentery	less	more

Fig. 4.14 Distinguishing characteristics of the jejunum and ileum.

The blood supply to the jejunum and ileum is from the jejunal and ileal branches of the superior mesenteric artery. The arteries form a series of anastomotic loops to make arterial arcades. From these arcades, straight arteries pass to the mesenteric border of the gut. The straight arteries are end arteries—occlusion may result in infarction.

Lymphatic drainage is to the superior mesenteric nodes.

Parasympathetic fibres from the vagus nerve increase peristalsis and secretion, whereas sympathetic fibres from the lateral horn of T9 and T10 inhibit peristalsis.

Large intestine

This consists of the caecum, appendix, colon, rectum, and anal canal.

Caecum and appendix

These lie in the right iliac fossa.

The caecum lies free in the abdominal cavity, invested by peritoneum. The ileum enters the caecum obliquely, and partially invaginates into it, forming the ileocaecal valve. The blood supply to the caecum is from the ileocolic artery.

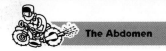

The appendix is a worm-shaped blind-ending tube with lymphoid tissue in its wall, and is usually 6–9 cm long. It opens into the posteromedial wall of the caecum, 2 cm below the ileocaecal valve. The appendix has its own mesentery, the mesoappendix.

Blood supply is from the appendicular artery, a branch of the posterior caecal artery. It is an end artery, and any swelling of the appendix may obstruct the artery, causing necrosis and perforation.

Appendicitis is a common surgical emergency. It usually presents with central abdominal pain, which later spreads to the right iliac fossa. The base of the appendix is usually identified externally at McBurney's point, one-third of the way along a line joining the anterior superior iliac spine and the umbilicus. Internally, the base of the appendix lies at the point of convergence of the taeniae coli.

Colon

Ascending colon

This extends from the ileocolic junction to the right colic (hepatic) flexure. On the medial and lateral sides of the ascending colon the peritoneum forms the paracolic gutters. Most of the colon has an incomplete longitudinal muscle layer represented by the three taeniae coli. Bulbous pouches of peritoneum distended with fat project from the serous coat. These are the appendices epiploicae.

Transverse colon

This extends from the right colic flexure to the left colic (splenic) flexure. It is completely invested in peritoneum and hangs free on the transverse mesocolon.

Descending colon

This extends from the splenic flexure to the pelvic brim. There are paracolic gutters on its medial and lateral sides.

Sigmoid colon

This extends from the descending colon to the pelvic brim. It hangs free from the sigmoid mesocolon, and where this mesentery ends, the rectum commences. In the terminal part of the sigmoid colon the three taeniae coli coalesce to form a complete longitudinal muscle layer.

The colon is supplied by the superior mesenteric artery (artery of the midgut) up to the proximal two-thirds of the transverse colon, and the inferior mesenteric artery thereafter (Fig. 4.15).

The branches anastomose near the medial margin of the entire colon, forming an arterial circle, the marginal artery, from which short vessels pass to the gut wall. The weakest part of the marginal artery supply to the colon is between the middle colic and left colic arteries at the splenic flexure. This site is thus most prone to ischaemia and infarction.

The venous drainage follows the arterial supply to the portal venous system.

The ascending and descending colons are held onto the posterior abdominal wall, i.e they are retroperitoneal. The transverse and sigmoid colons are suspended by mesenteries and are mobile.

Spleen

This is a large lymphoid organ. It removes particulate matter and aged or defective cells from the circulation and helps in mounting an immunological response against blood-borne pathogens. The importance of the spleen as an immunological organ is emphasized in people, particularly children, who have their spleens removed. These patients are very susceptible to infections by encapsulated organisms such as the pneumococcus and meningococcus, both of which may cause fatal meningitis. These individuals often need antibiotics life long to prevent infection, together with vaccinations.

The spleen lies deep to the 9th to 11th ribs and has a convex diaphragmatic surface that fits into the concavity of the diaphragm. The anterior and superior borders are notched and sharp, but the posterior and inferior borders are rounded.

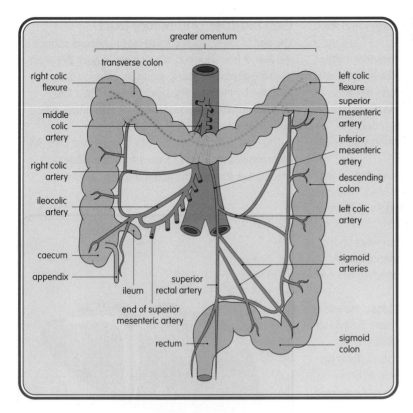

Fig. 4.15 Colon and its blood supply.

Labels in figure:
- greater omentum
- transverse colon
- right colic flexure
- left colic flexure
- superior mesenteric artery
- middle colic artery
- inferior mesenteric artery
- right colic artery
- descending colon
- ileocolic artery
- left colic artery
- caecum
- sigmoid arteries
- appendix
- superior rectal artery
- ileum
- end of superior mesenteric artery
- rectum
- sigmoid colon

The spleen contacts the posterior wall of the stomach. It is connected to the greater curvature of the stomach by the gastrosplenic ligament and to the posterior abdominal wall at the left kidney by the splenorenal ligament. It is completely enclosed by peritoneum except at the hilum.

The splenic artery from the coeliac trunk is a tortuous vessel that passes along the superior border of the pancreas and anterior to the left kidney. Between the layers of the splenorenal ligament, the splenic artery divides into five or more branches, which enter the hilum.

The splenic vein joins the inferior mesenteric vein and runs posterior to the body of the pancreas to unite with the superior mesenteric vein to form the hepatic portal vein.

Lymphatic drainage is to the pancreaticosplenic and coeliac nodes.

The spleen is very susceptible to abdominal trauma and may bleed profusely, resulting in collapse of the patient and shock. Emergency splenectomy may be life saving in these cases.

The spleen is a foregut derivative.

Liver

The liver is a wedge-shaped organ lying in the right hypochondrium. It is largely under cover of the costal margin and is invested by peritoneum except over its bare area.

The liver has four lobes (Fig. 4.16). The falciform ligament divides the liver into right and left lobes. Posteriorly there is also a caudate lobe lying between the inferior vena cava and the ligamentum venosum fissure, and a quadrate lobe lying between the gall bladder fossa and the ligamentum teres. Functionally, the quadrate and caudate lobes are part of the left lobe as they are supplied by the left hepatic artery and left bile duct.

The falciform ligament runs up the anterior surface of the liver. At the superior surface of the liver the left leaf passes to the left and returns to form the left triangular ligament. The right leaf forms the upper leaf of the coronary ligament, the right triangular ligament, and the lower leaf of the coronary ligament (Fig. 4.16).

The area between the upper and lower parts of the coronary ligament is the bare area of the liver. This area is devoid of peritoneum and lies in contact with the diaphragm.

The right and left layers of peritoneum meet on the visceral surface of the liver to form the hepatogastric and hepatoduodenal ligaments, both of which are part of the lesser omentum.

Between the caudate and quadrate lobes, the two layers surround the porta hepatis. This, with the inferior vena cava, the gall bladder, and the fissures of the ligamentum venosum and ligamentum teres, form an H-shaped pattern. The ligamentum venosum is the remnant of the fetal ductus venosus, which transported blood from the portal and umbilical veins to the hepatic veins.

The porta hepatis contains the right and left branches of the hepatic artery, the hepatic ducts, and the hepatic portal vein (Fig. 4.16):

- The hepatic artery from the coeliac trunk supplies oxygenated blood to the lobes of the liver. The cystic artery arises from it to supply the gall bladder.
- The hepatic portal vein carries the products of digestion from the gut to the liver.
- The right and left hepatic ducts drain bile into the common hepatic duct. The latter joins the cystic duct to form the bile duct.

There are also three hepatic veins that drain the liver. These do not have an extrahepatic course but drain directly into the inferior vena cava.

Lymphatics drain into the hepatic nodes lying around the porta hepatis. They also drain the gall bladder. The hepatic nodes drain into the coeliac nodes. Lymphatics of the bare area drain into the posterior mediastinal nodes.

Nerve supply is from the left vagus nerve and the sympathetic coeliac ganglion.

Gall bladder and biliary tract

The gall bladder lies in a fossa on the visceral surface of the liver. It has a fundus, a body, and a neck (Fig. 4.17).

The gall bladder stores and concentrates bile secreted by the liver. The bile is released into the duodenum when the gall bladder is stimulated, e.g. after a fatty meal.

The cystic duct drains the gall bladder and joins the common hepatic duct to form the common bile duct. This passes through the free margin of the lesser

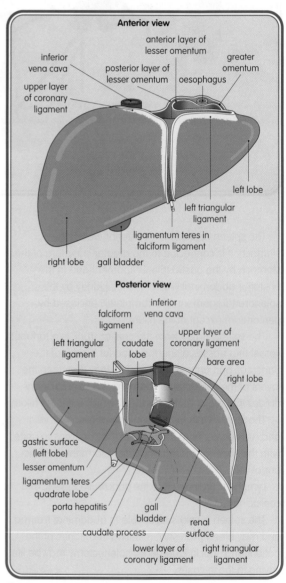

Fig. 4.16 Anterior and posterior views of the liver.

omentum behind the first part of the duodenum to enter the second part of the duodenum, together with the pancreatic duct, at the hepatopancreatic ampulla (of Vater). The sphincter of Oddi is a layer of circular muscle surrounding the ampulla. It controls the flow of bile and pancreatic secretions into the duodenum. The mucosa lining the neck and cystic duct is thrown into folds to form a spiral valve.

Obstruction of the biliary system results in the clinical condition of jaundice (yellow skin).

Also, the gall bladder is prone to accumulating gallstones. These may pass into the duct system, causing severe colicky pain (biliary colic).

Blood supply is from the cystic artery, a branch of the hepatic artery. Numerous branches from the hepatic bed also supply the gall bladder.

Pancreas

The pancreas has both exocrine and endocrine functions. It lies behind the peritoneum on the posterior abdominal wall, roughly at the level of the transpyloric plane (see Fig. 4.13). It has a head, neck, body, and tail:

- The head lies in the concavity of the duodenum, anterior to the inferior vena cava and left renal vein. The bile duct travels through it. A small part of the head, the uncinate process, lies behind the superior mesenteric artery and vein.
- The neck overlies the superior mesenteric vessels and the portal vein.
- The body crosses the left renal vein and the aorta. The splenic vessels run close to this part of the pancreas.
- The tail is accompanied by the splenic vessels and lymphatics in the lienorenal (splenorenal) ligament, to touch the hilum of the spleen.

The main pancreatic duct opens into the duodenum with the bile duct, at the ampulla of Vater. The accessory duct opens into the duodenum 2 cm proximal to the ampulla of Vater.

The splenic artery, a branch of the coeliac trunk, supplies the neck, body, and tail of the pancreas. The superior and inferior pancreaticoduodenal arteries supply the head. The splenic vein drains the pancreas. Lymphatics drain into the coeliac and superior mesenteric nodes.

Carcinoma of the pancreas has a very poor prognosis, probably because it is silent and asymptomatic for a long time. If the head of the pancreas is involved, the bile duct running through it may become blocked, leading to jaundice. This may alert the clinician sooner.

Vessels of the gut

The foregut, midgut, and hindgut are supplied by the branches of the coeliac trunk, the superior mesenteric artery, and the inferior mesenteric artery, respectively.

The coeliac trunk arises from the abdominal aorta at the level of T12 vertebra. It gives off the left gastric artery, the hepatic artery, and the splenic artery (see Fig. 4.12).

The superior mesenteric artery arises from the abdominal aorta at the level of L1 vertebra (transpyloric plane). It gives off the inferior pancreaticoduodenal artery, jejunal and ileal arteries, and the ileocolic, right colic, and middle colic arteries (see Fig. 4.15).

The inferior mesenteric artery arises from the abdominal aorta, opposite L3 vertebra. It gives off the left colic artery, sigmoid arteries, and the superior rectal artery (see Fig. 4.15).

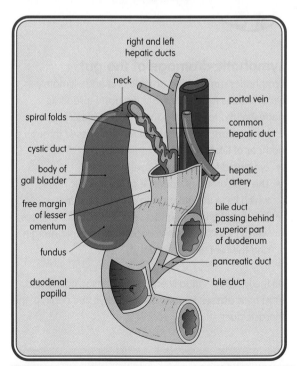

Fig. 4.17 Gallbladder and biliary tract. (Adapted from *Anatomy as a Basis for Clinical Medicine*, by E.C.B. Hall-Craggs. Courtesy of Williams & Wilkins.)

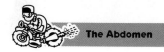

Venous drainage of the gut

Venous blood rich in nutrients from the intestines travels in the hepatic portal system of veins to the liver (Fig. 4.18). From the liver the blood passes to the inferior vena cava via the hepatic veins and then to the heart.

Portosystemic anastomoses

These are areas with both a portal and a systemic venous drainage. They include the oesophagus, the anal canal, the retroperitoneum and the umbilical region. The most significant of these is the oesophagus.

Portal hypertension caused by liver diseases obstructs portal blood flow and blood is diverted to the systemic veins. This increased volume through the systemic veins causes them to dilate, forming varices. These may rupture if traumatized, causing severe haemorrhage and even death.

Nerve supply of the gastrointestinal tract

All parts of the gut receive sympathetic and parasympathetic nerves that travel with the gut arteries. Sympathetic fibres come from the sympathetic chain and from the coeliac, superior mesenteric, and inferior mesenteric plexuses. Parasympathetic fibres for the foregut and midgut enter the abdomen in the vagus nerves and are distributed either directly or via the coeliac and superior mesenteric plexuses. Parasympathetic supply to the hindgut ascends from the pelvis (S2–S4) in the hypogastric plexus. .

Sympathetic fibres inhibit peristalsis and secretion; parasympathetic fibres increase them.

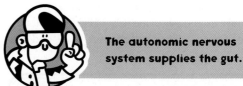

The autonomic nervous system supplies the gut.

Lymphatic drainage of the gut

Lymphatics run with the arteries and end ultimately in lymph nodes lying anterior to the aorta (preaortic nodes) at the roots of the three gut arteries.

Lymph from the mucosa of the gut passes through a number of filters including:

- Lymphoid follicles, e.g. Peyer's patches.
- The 'epi' group of nodes, e.g. the epicolic nodes, which lie in the gut margin of the mesentery.
- The 'para' group of nodes, e.g. the paracolic nodes, which lie in the mesentery between the gut margin and the root of the mesentery.

All the lymph eventually enters the coeliac nodes and from here passes into the cisterna chyli, the origin of the thoracic duct.

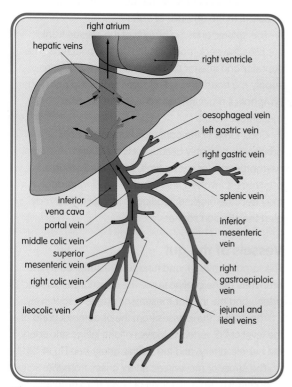

Fig. 4.18 Hepatic portal venous system. (Adapted from *Anatomy as a Basis for Clinical Medicine*, by E.C.B. Hall-Craggs. Courtesy of Williams & Wilkins.)

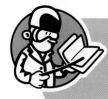

- Outline the anatomy of the abdominal organs.
- Discuss the blood supply of the gut.
- Describe the nerve supply of the abdominal cavity.
- Describe the lymphatic drainage of the abdominal cavity.

THE POSTERIOR ABDOMINAL WALL

The posterior abdominal wall offers good protection to the abdominal contents. It is composed of the bodies of the five lumbar vertebrae and their intervertebral discs, and the psoas, iliacus, and quadratus lumborum muscles.

The lumbar vertebrae project forwards into the abdominal cavity with a forward convexity (lumbar lordosis). The inferior vena cava and the aorta lie in front of the bodies of the vertebrae.

On either side of the vertebral bodies lie the paravertebral gutters. The kidneys and suprarenal glands lie in the superior aspect of these gutters (Fig. 4.19).

Muscles of the posterior abdominal wall

These are outlined in Fig. 4.20.

Fascia of the posterior abdominal wall

The muscles of the posterior abdominal wall are covered by thick, strong fascia, which provide firm support for the peritoneum and retroperitoneal viscera.

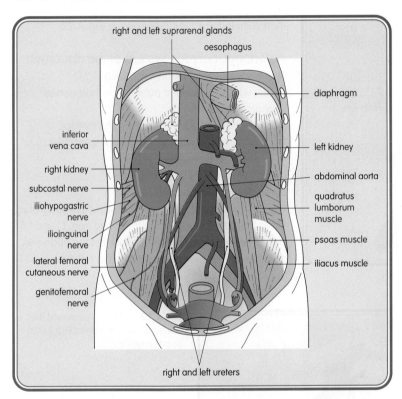

Fig. 4.19 Structures of the posterior abdominal wall.

Fig. 4.20 Muscles of the posterior abdominal wall. (Adapted from *Clinical Anatomy, An Illustrated Review with Questions and Explanations 2e*, by R.S. Snell. Courtesy of Churchill Livingstone.)

Muscles of the posterior abdominal wall			
Name of muscle (nerve supply)	Origin	Insertion	Action
psoas (lumbar plexus)	transverse process, bodies, and intervertebral discs of T12 and L1–L5 vertebrae	lesser trochanter of femur	flexes thigh on trunk
quadratus lumborum (lumbar plexus)	iliolumbar ligament, iliac crest, transverse processes of lower lumbar vertebrae	12th rib	depresses 12th rib during respiration; laterally flexes vertebral column
iliacus (femoral nerve)	iliac fossa	lesser trochanter of femur	flexes thigh on trunk

Vessels of the posterior abdominal wall
Abdominal aorta

The abdominal aorta passes through the diaphragm at the level of T12 vertebra. It passes inferiorly on the bodies of the lumbar vertebrae. In front of the body of L4 it divides into the common iliac arteries (Fig. 4.21).

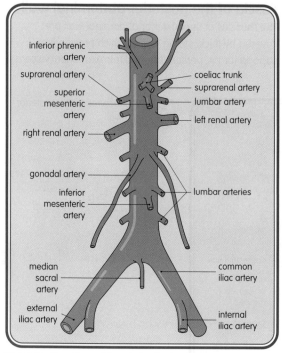

Fig. 4.21 Branches of the abdominal aorta.

Inferior vena cava

This vessel is formed on the right side of the aortic bifurcation, by the union of the two common iliac veins (see Fig. 3.22). It ascends to the right of the aorta and passes behind the liver to pierce the diaphragm at the level of T8 vertebra and almost immediately enters the heart.

Nerves of the posterior abdominal wall
Somatic nerves

The lumbar spinal nerves emerge from the intervertebral foramina and pass into the psoas muscle. They supply this muscle and quadratus lumborum, and then unite to form the lumbar plexus (Fig. 4.22)

Autonomic nervous system of the abdomen

This is composed of the following (Fig. 4.23):
- The vagus nerves and pelvic splanchnic nerves (parasympathetic).
- The lumbar sympathetic trunks, the thoracic splanchnic nerves, and the lumbar splanchnic nerves (sympathetic).

Sympathetic nerves

The lumbar sympathetic trunk comprises preganglionic fibres from the lower thoracic trunk and from L1 and L2 nerves (via white rami). This trunk enters the abdomen posterior to the medial arcuate ligament of the

Fig. 4.22 Lumbar plexus and the relationship of the branches to the psoas muscle.

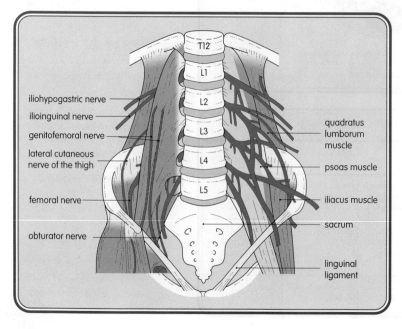

diaphragm. It runs down on the medial border of psoas major.

There are usually four lumbar ganglia. These give somatic branches (grey rami communicantes) to all five lumbar nerves, supplying the body wall and lower limb, and visceral branches (lumbar splanchnic nerves) that join the coeliac, aortic, and superior hypogastric plexuses. Fibres from the third and fourth ganglia join with fibres from the aortic plexus in front of L5 vertebra to form the superior hypogastric plexus. The superior hypogastric plexus divides into the right and left hypogastric nerves. These run into the pelvis to join the inferior hypogastric plexus. There are no branches to the abdominal viscera.

The greater and lesser splanchnic nerves pierce the crura of the diaphragm to enter the coeliac ganglion. These splanchnic nerves are almost totally preganglionic and relay in the coeliac ganglia. The least splanchnic nerves relay in a small renal ganglion close to the renal artery.

From the coeliac ganglion, postganglionic fibres form a rich network around the aorta, the coeliac plexus. This is situated around the origin of the coeliac trunk and supplies all the abdominal viscera via the visceral branches of the aorta. Fibres passing to the kidneys pick up branches from the renal ganglion to form the renal plexus around the renal artery.

The suprarenal gland has a second supply in addition to the coeliac plexus. Preganglionic fibres from the lesser splanchnic nerve pass without relay to the cells of the suprarenal medulla. Stimulation causes the release of adrenaline.

Functions of the sympathetic nerves include vasomotor, motor to the sphincters, inhibition of peristalsis, and transport of sensory fibres from all of the abdominal viscera.

Parasympathetic nerves

The vagal trunks enter the abdomen on the surface of the oesophagus. Branches to the coeliac plexus supply the gut up to the transverse colon. Branches to the renal plexus pass to the kidneys. The distal part of the transverse colon and the descending and sigmoid colons receive parasympathetic innervation from the pelvic splanchnic nerves.

Functions of the parasympathetic nerves comprise motor and secretomotor to the gut and glands.

Kidneys

These organs lie largely under cover of the costal margin in the paravertebral gutters of the posterior abdominal wall. The position of the kidneys varies with respiration, but they lie approximately opposite the first three lumbar vertebrae. The right kidney is lower than the left kidney, as it lies below the liver (Fig. 4.24).

Each kidney is surrounded by perinephric fat. The renal fascia encloses these two structures and separates the kidney from the suprarenal gland. The fascia is firmly attached to the renal vessels and the ureter at the hilum of the kidney.

A renal artery supplies each kidney (Fig. 4.25). At the hilum of the kidney the main artery divides into anterior and posterior branches. These are further subdivided into segmental arteries and then into interlobular arteries. Venous drainage is via the renal vein.

Ureters

The ureters are formed at the renal pelvis. They descend on the psoas muscle behind the peritoneum and cross the common iliac artery at its bifurcation at the pelvic brim. They turn towards the bladder at the level of the ischial spine.

Fig. 4.23 Autonomic nerves and plexuses of the abdomen.

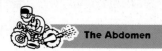
The ureter narrows in three places:
- At the pelvoureteric junction.
- Where it crosses the pelvic brim.
- At its termination in the bladder.

Blood supply is from the renal artery, the abdominal aorta, the gonadal and vesical arteries, the common and internal iliac arteries, and the middle rectal artery.

Carcinoma of the cervix is a very common tumour in middle-aged women. Advanced cases may cause renal failure by obstructing the ureters and are often fatal.

Suprarenal gland

This gland lies on the medial aspect of the superior pole of each kidney. It is separated from the kidney by the renal fascia. The suprarenal gland secretes several hormones (e.g. corticosteroids, adrenaline) which are essential for life. It consists of a central medulla and a peripheral cortex.

The suprarenal gland is supplied by three main vessels:
- The suprarenal branch of the inferior phrenic artery.
- The suprarenal branch of the renal artery.
- The suprarenal artery.

Lymph from the kidneys and the suprarenal glands drains into the para-aortic lymph nodes.

- Describe the anatomy of the kidney and suprarenal gland.
- Discuss the vessels and nerves of the posterior abdominal wall.

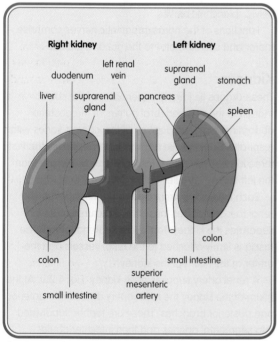

Fig. 4.24 Kidneys and their main anterior relations.

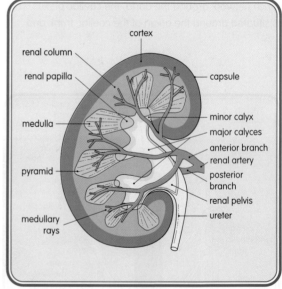

Fig. 4.25 Macroscopic structure and arterial supply of the kidney.

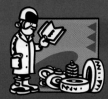

5. The Pelvis and Perineum

REGIONS AND COMPONENTS OF THE PELVIS

The pelvis lies below and behind the abdomen and is where the trunk communicates with the lower limbs. It is enclosed by bony, muscular, and ligamentous walls.

The bony pelvis is formed by the two hip bones and the sacrum and coccyx. It has an upper part, the greater pelvis, flanked by the iliac bones, and a lower part, the lesser pelvis. The greater and lesser pelves meet at the pelvic brim (Fig. 5.1).

The pelvic cavity is continuous with the abdominal cavity and is therefore lined by the peritoneum of the greater peritoneal sac. The peritoneum passes down into the pelvis to cover partially the terminal portions of the alimentary tract, the bladder, and the internal reproductive organs of the female.

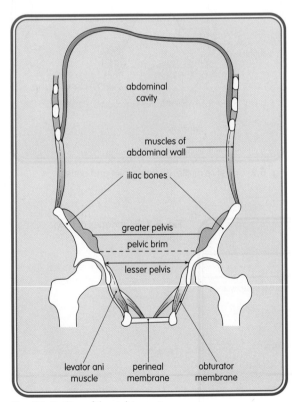

Fig. 5.1 Outline of the pelvic cavity.

The contents of the pelvis include:
- The rectum and sigmoid colon.
- The ureters and bladder.
- The ovaries, fallopian tubes, uterus, and vagina in females.
- The ductus deferens, seminal vesicles, and prostate in males.
- The lumbosacral trunk, obturator nerve, sympathetic trunks, and sacral plexus.
- The common iliac arteries, gonadal arteries, and superior rectal arteries.

SURFACE ANATOMY AND SUPERFICIAL STRUCTURES

Bony landmarks

The iliac crest can be felt along its entire length. The anterior superior iliac spine is at the anterior border of the iliac crest and lies in the fold of the groin superiorly. The posterior superior iliac spine is at the posterior end of the iliac crest. It lies under a skin dimple at the level of S2 vertebra.

The pubic tubercle can be felt on the upper border of the pubis. The symphysis pubis joins the two pubic bones and may also be palpated. The pubic crest is a ridge of bone on the superior surface of the pubic bone, medial to the pubic tubercle.

The spinous processes of the sacrum fuse to form the median sacral crest. The crest can be felt beneath the skin in the buttock cleft. The sacral hiatus is found at the lower end of the sacrum, about 5 cm above the coccyx. The coccyx may be palpated about 2.5 cm behind the anus.

Viscera

The bladder is a pelvic organ in the adult, but when full may be palpated through the anterior abdominal wall. The non-pregnant uterus is not usually palpable. In pregnancy the fundus of the uterus may be palpated from about week 12. At term the fundus is usually at the level of the xiphisternum.

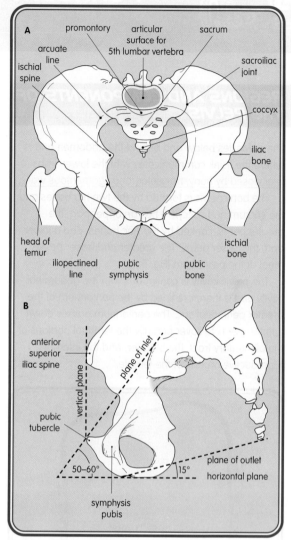

Fig. 5.2 (A) Pelvic girdle. (B) Pelvic inlet and outlet.

○ Describe the surface anatomy of the pelvis.

THE BONY PELVIS AND PELVIC WALL

Bony pelvis

The bony pelvis is formed by the two hip bones, the sacrum, and the coccyx (Fig. 5.2). The hip bones meet anteriorly at the pubic symphysis; posteriorly they articulate with the sacrum at the sacroiliac joints. The bony pelvis thus forms a ring that protects the pelvic contents.

The pelvis is divided into the greater pelvis (false pelvis), which lies above the pelvic brim (pelvic inlet), and the lesser pelvis, which lies between the pelvic inlet and pelvic outlet (Fig. 5.3). The pelvic inlet lies at about 45 degrees to the pelvic outlet.

Sacrum

The sacrum consists of the fused five sacral vertebrae (Fig. 5.4). There are anterior and posterior sacral foramina for passage of the anterior and posterior rami of the sacral spinal nerves. The median sacral crest represents the fused spinal processes of the sacral vertebrae.

Fig. 5.3 Boundaries of pelvic apertures.

Boundaries of pelvic apertures	
Pelvic inlet	**Pelvic outlet**
superior border of the pubic symphysis	inferior margin of the pubic symphysis
posterior border of the pubic crest	inferior ramus of the pubis and the ischial tuberosity
pecten of the pubis	
arcuate line of the ilium	sacrotuberous ligaments
anterior border of the ala of the sacrum	tip of the coccyx
sacral promontory	

The sacrum articulates with the hip bone via its articular surface at the sacroiliac joints.

Hip bone

This is formed by the fusion of the ilium, the ischium, and the pubic bone shortly after puberty (Fig. 5.5).

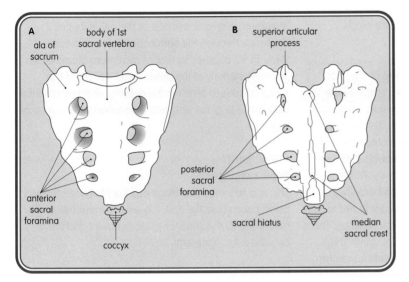

Fig. 5.4 (A) Anterior and (B) posterior views of the sacrum.

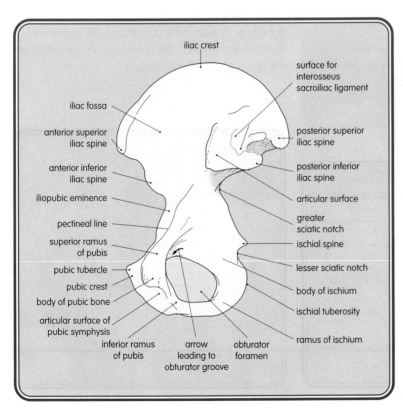

Fig. 5.5 Medial view of the hip bone.

Ilium

The iliac fossa gives rise to the iliacus muscle, and the articular surface forms the sacroiliac joint. The iliac crest, and the anterior superior and posterior superior iliac spines lie superiorly. There are also anterior inferior and posterior inferior iliac spines (see Fig. 5.5)

The ilium contributes to the formation of the acetabulum and the bony margin of the greater sciatic notch.

Pubis and ischium

The pubic bones articulate in the midline at the pubic symphysis (see Fig. 5.5). On the upper surface of the body are the pubic crest and pubic tubercle. Each pubic bone has a superior and inferior ramus. The superior ramus forms the superior border of the obturator foramen. The inferior ramus unites the pubis with the ischial bone to form the ischiopubic ramus. This leads to the body of the ischium and the ischial tuberosity.

The posterior border of the ischium contributes to the formation of the greater and lesser sciatic notches. The two notches are separated by the ischial spine. The sacrotuberous and sacrospinous ligaments transform the notches into the greater and lesser sciatic foramina.

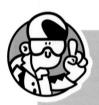

The three bones of the hip all contribute to the formation of the acetabulum.

Male and female pelves

The male and female pelves may show a great deal of sexual dimorphism (Fig. 5.6).

The largest diameter of the pelvic inlet is the transverse diameter (Fig. 5.7), while the largest diameter of the pelvic outlet is the anteroposterior diameter. As the foetal head enters the pelvic inlet its maximum diameter lies across the pelvis, but as it descends through the birth canal the head rotates through 90 degrees so that its maximum diameter lies anteroposteriorly at the pelvic outlet. Failure of this rotation leads to arrest in the delivery, and instrumental assistance (e.g. forceps) or a caesarean section may be required.

Pelvic joints

Pubic symphysis

This is a secondary cartilaginous joint between the two pubic bones (see Fig. 5.5). It is usually immobile and is reinforced by the superior pubic ligament and the arcuate pubic ligament.

Sacroiliac joint

This is a synovial joint, but it allows only minimal movement. It is strengthened by strong interosseous ligaments. Weaker anterior and posterior ligaments also stabilize the joint. The joint transmits the weight of the upper body to the hip bones.

Differences between the male and female pelves		
	Male	**Female**
acetabulum	large	small
build	robust	thin
inferior pelvic aperture	relatively small	relatively large
obturator foramen	round	oval
pubic arch	narrow	wide
superior pelvic aperture	usually heart-shaped	usually oval or rounded

Fig. 5.6 Differences between the male and female pelves.

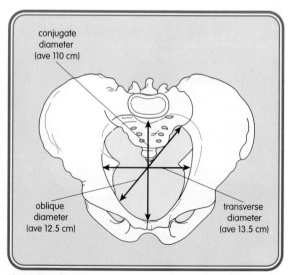

Fig. 5.7 Pelvic inlet and its diameters. (ave, average.)

Pelvic wall and floor

The side wall of the pelvis is formed by the hip bone with the obturator internus muscle (Fig. 5.8). The posterior wall is formed by the sacrum and the piriformis muscle as it passes into the greater sciatic foramen.

The pelvic floor forms a gutter of muscle around the terminal parts of the rectum and the prostate and urethra in the male and the vagina and urethra in the female (Fig. 5.9).

Fig. 5.10 outlines the muscles of the pelvic wall and floor.

Perineal body

This is a midline knot of fibromuscular tissue lying posterior to the prostate or vagina. Parts of the levator ani and the external sphincter of the anal canal are fused with it.

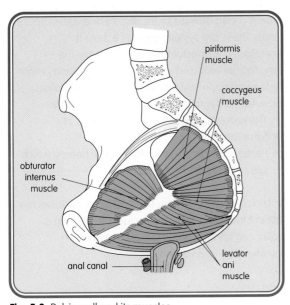

Fig. 5.8 Pelvic wall and its muscles.

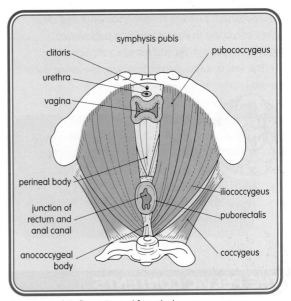

Fig. 5.9 Pelvic floor viewed from below.

Muscles of the pelvic wall and floor			
Name of muscle (nerve supply)	**Origin**	**Insertion**	**Action**
coccygeus (4th and 5th sacral nerves)	ischial spine	inferior aspect of sacrum and coccyx	supports pelvic viscera, flexes coccyx
levator ani (pudendal nerve, 4th sacral nerve)	ischial spine body of pubis fascia of obturator internus	perineal body anococcygeal body walls of prostate, vagina, rectum, and anal canal	supports pelvic viscera; sphincter to anorectal junction and vagina counteracts increased abdominal pressure, e.g. defaecation, parturition
piriformis (sacral plexus)	anterior aspect of sacrum	greater trochanter of femur	rotates femur laterally at hip
obturator internus (sacral plexus)	obturator membrane and adjacent hip bone	greater trochanter of femur	rotates femur laterally at hip

Fig. 5.10 Muscles of the pelvic wall and floor.

Damage to the perineal body during childbirth may result in prolapse of the bladder, vagina, and uterus.

Pelvic fascia

Over the pelvic wall the fascia is a strong membrane covering the obturator internus and piriformis muscles. The spinal nerves lie external to the fascia and the vessels lie internal to it. The sacral plexus lies betwen the fascia and the piriformis muscles.

Over the pelvic floor the fascia consists of loose areolar tissue. The fascia condenses around the neurovascular bundles to form ligaments and also gives rise to the puboprostatic and pubovesical ligaments in the male and female, respectively.

The fascia varies in thickness over the pelvic viscera.

- Describe the main features of the bones and joints of the pelvis.
- Discuss the muscles of the pelvic floor and wall.

THE PELVIC CONTENTS

Pelvic organs

Rectum

The rectum commences as a continuation of the sigmoid colon (where the sigmoid mesocolon ends) at the level of the third piece of the sacrum. It ends at the anorectal junction by piercing the pelvic floor at the border of the puborectalis muscle to become the anal canal.

The rectum has three lateral curves and its lowest part dilates as the rectal ampulla. There are also three transverse folds containing both mucous membrane and circular muscle.

The rectum has no mesentery. Peritoneum covers the upper third of the rectum at the front and sides, and the middle third of the rectum at the front. The lower third lies below the level of the peritoneum, and the latter is reflected onto the bladder or vagina to form the rectovesical or rectouterine pouch (of Douglas). These pouches are the lowest parts of the peritoneal cavity and are filled with small bowel and the sigmoid colon (Fig. 5.11)

Posteriorly the rectum is related to the sacrum, coccyx, and pelvic floor.

Vessels and nerves of the rectum

Blood supply is from the superior, middle, and inferior rectal arteries. The superior rectal artery is a continuation of the inferior mesenteric artery. The others are discussed in the section describing the blood supply to the pelvis.

The rectal plexus of veins drains into the inferior mesenteric vein (portal system of veins). The rectal plexus is also drained by the middle and inferior rectal veins. These are systemic veins, i.e there is portosystemic anastomosis in the rectum. The longitudinal venous channels of the rectum may dilate to form haemorrhoids. Unlike oesophageal varices, however, this is rarely due to to portal obstruction.

The nerve supply of the rectum consists of:
- Sympathetic—hypogastric plexus.
- Parasympathetic—pelvic splanchnic nerves, which are motor to the rectal muscles.

In Hirschsprung's disease the autonomic plexuses are absent from the wall of the rectum. The rectum is collapsed and this leads to bowel obstruction, constipation, and vomiting.

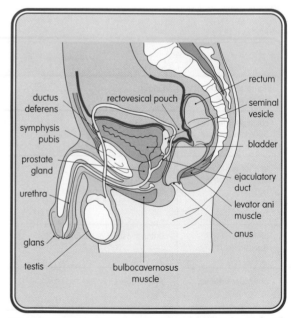

Fig. 5.11 Sagittal section through the male pelvis, illustrating the rectum and rectovesical pouch.

Lymphatics accompany branches of the superior and middle rectal arteries and eventually drain to the preaortic nodes at the origin of the inferior mesenteric vessels.

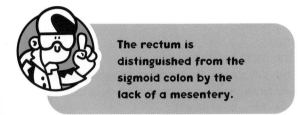

The rectum is distinguished from the sigmoid colon by the lack of a mesentery.

Ureters in the pelvis

The ureters cross the pelvic brim at the bifurcation of the common iliac vessels (Fig. 5.12). They continue into the lesser pelvis towards the ischial spines and cross the obturator nerve and vessels. At the pelvic floor they run forward to enter the base of the bladder near its superior angle. Here, in males, the ductus deferens crosses the ureter superiorly; in females, the uterine artery crosses the ureter.

The ureter may be damaged in hysterectomy (removal of the uterus) when it may be tied while attempting to tie off the uterine artery.

Bladder

The undistended bladder is a pyramid-shaped organ (Fig. 5.13). The apex points towards the pubic symphysis and the median umbilical ligament is attached to it.

The base is triangular. In males it lies largely below the rectovesical pouch and is not covered by peritoneum. The ductus deferens and the seminal vesicles are attached to the surface and the ureter enters the bladder at its superolateral surface. In females the base is firmly attached to the vaginal wall and the upper part of the cervix by connective tissue.

Two inferolateral surfaces become continuous with each other at the retropubic space.

The bladder is composed of smooth muscle, the detrusor muscle, in an interlacing network of fibres running in several directions. This gives the bladder its trabeculated appearance and is supplied by the parasympathetic nerves.

The urethra leaves the bladder at its inferior angle. The smooth muscle of the bladder is arranged in a circular fashion around the commencement of the urethra, the sphincter vesicae.

Internal surface of the bladder

When the bladder is empty, the mucosa is thick and folded. As the bladder fills, the mucosa becomes thinner and smoother.

Fig. 5.12 Course of the ureter in the pelvis of the male.

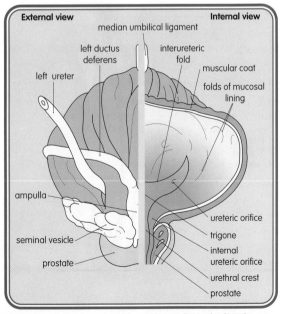

Fig. 5.13 Base of the bladder in the male and related structures.

The trigone is a triangular area lying between the urethral orifice and the two ureteric orifices. It is the least mobile part of the bladder and the mucosa here is always smooth. The interureteric fold connects the two ureteric orifices.

The ureters pierce the mucosa obliquely, and the valve-like flap of mucosa produced is important in preventing reflux of urine when intravesical pressure increases. The ureteric orifices are closed by this pressure and opened by peristaltic activity. Abnormal insertion of the ureters in the bladder may lead to reflux of urine up the ureters and even to the kidneys. This is a common problem in children and may result in hypertension and renal failure.

Vessels and nerves of the bladder

Blood supply is from the superior and inferior vesical arteries, with minor contributions from the obturator, uterine, inferior gluteal, and vaginal arteries.

In males, veins form the vesicoprostatic plexus, which drain into the internal iliac veins. A similar plexus is formed in females.

The nerve supply comprises:
- Parasympathetic (motor)—pelvic splanchnic nerves.
- Sympathetic—the superior hypogastric and pelvic plexuses.

The male urethra

This is 20 cm long, commencing at the bladder neck and terminating at the external urethral orifice (Fig. 5.14). It has three parts:
- The prostatic urethra has an elevated central region on its posterior wall, the urethral crest. The crest expands to form the seminal colliculus on which lies the prostatic utricle. The orifices of the ejaculatory ducts open on either side of this.

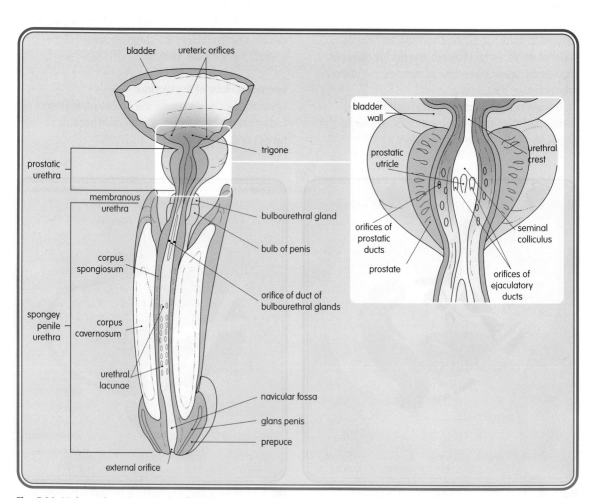

Fig. 5.14 Male urethra (showing details of the prostatic urethra).

- The membranous urethra lies between the apex of the prostate and the bulb of the penis. It is surrounded by the sphincter urethrae and the perineal membrane. The bulbourethral glands lie on either side of it.
- The spongy urethra passes through the bulb, corpus spongiosum, and glans of the penis. Immediately before the external urethral orifice, the urethra expands to form the navicular fossa.

Numerous urethral glands open throughout the course of the urethra.

The female urethra

This is only 4 cm long. It runs from the bladder neck, through the pelvic floor and the perineal membrane, to open into the vestibule, anterior to the vaginal opening.

The female urethra, being shorter than that of the male, is more prone to urinary tract infections by ascending organisms.

Male reproductive organs in the pelvis

Ductus deferens

This passes from the epididymis to the pelvic cavity via the inguinal canal. At the deep inguinal ring it hooks around the inferior epigastric artery, crossing the external iliac vessels to enter the pelvic cavity. It crosses the obturator neurovascular bundle and the ureter to reach the base of the bladder (see Fig. 5.13). The terminal part dilates, forming the ampulla, and joins the duct of the seminal vesicle to form the ejaculatory duct, which opens into the prostatic urethra on the colliculus.

Seminal vesicles

These are two structures lying lateral to the ampulla of the ductus deferens (see Fig. 5.13).

Prostate gland

This is a chestnut-shaped organ that lies below the bladder and above the urogenital diaphragm (see Fig. 5.14). It has a base that is attached to the bladder and an apex that points inferiorly.

The prostate has right and left lobes united by an isthmus. The median lobe lies above and behind the lateral lobes and receives the ejaculatory ducts.

The prostate is pierced by the proximal urethra.

The capsule of the prostate completely surrounds the gland, and a thick sheath of pelvic fascia surrounds the capsule. The two are separated by the prostatic plexus of veins.

Blood supply is from the inferior vesical artery. Veins drain to the prostatic plexus, which eventually drains into the internal iliac veins.

Prostatic enlargement affects almost all elderly males. It may cause urinary obstruction. The enlargement may be due to a benign lesion or a prostatic carcinoma.

Semen produced by the seminal vesicles and prostate is added to the spermatozoa delivered to the urethra. A single ejaculate is about 3.0 mL.

The female reproductive tract

Uterus

This is a muscular organ that accommodates the developing embryo. Most of the wall is smooth muscle, the myometrium. The mucosa is the endometrium.

The uterus has three parts (Fig. 5.15):
- The fundus lies above the entrance of the fallopian tube.
- The body receives the fallopian tubes. It is enclosed by peritoneum, which laterally becomes the broad ligament. The cavity of the uterus occupies the body.
- The cervix is the narrowest part of the uterus. It has a supravaginal part and a vaginal part. The vaginal fornix surrounds the cervix, deepest posteriorly. The cervical canal is continuous with the uterine cavity at the internal os. It opens into the vagina at the external os.

The cervical canal is lined by columnar epithelium; the vagina is lined by stratified squamous epithelium. Between the two regions is a transition zone where cervical carcinomas arise. A cervical smear attempts to identify premalignant lesions so they can be removed before cancers arise.

The upper anterior, superior, and posterior surfaces of the uterus are covered by peritoneum. Posteriorly the peritoneum is reflected onto the rectum to form the rectouterine pouch (Fig. 5.16). The peritoneum continues from the lateral surface of the uterus to the pelvic side wall as the broad ligament.

Fallopian (uterine) tubes

These extend from the junction of the body and fundus of the uterus. They run in the upper edge of the broad ligament (see Fig. 5.15). The peritoneum investing each tube is the mesosalpinx.

The fallopian tube is composed of the isthmus, the ampulla, and the infundibulum. The outer end of the infundibulum is fimbriated. One of these fimbria, the ovarian fimbria, is attached to the ovary.

When the ovum is shed into the peritoneal cavity, it is taken up by the infundibulum and passed to the uterus.

Fertilization usually occurs in the tubes, but occasionally the fertilized ovum may implant in the tube (an ectopic pregnancy).

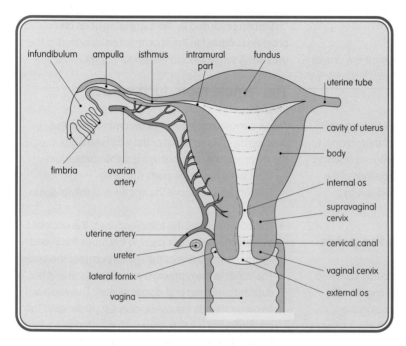

Fig. 5.15 Uterus and its blood supply.

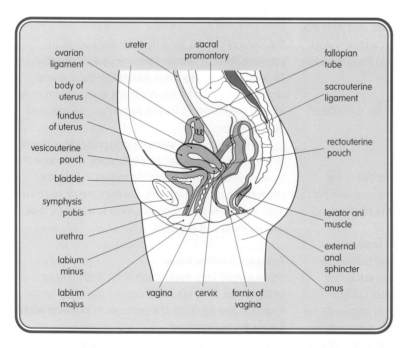

Fig. 5.16 Sagittal section through the female pelvis.

Ligaments of the uterus

The broad ligament is a double fold of peritoneum that is attached to the uterus and pelvic side wall (Fig. 5.17). It forms the mesosalpinx for the uterine tubes and the mesovarium for the ovary.

The suspensory ligament of the ovary contains the ovarian vessels and lymphatics. The anterior layer of the broad ligament is pushed forward by the round ligament of the uterus. The posterior layer bulges backwards as the mesovarium, suspending the ovary.

The round ligament extends from the body of the uterus to the pelvic brim. It passes through the inguinal canal to the labium majus. It is the remnant of the gubernaculum (see Testis, p. 62).

Transverse cervical ligaments (cardinal ligaments) are thickened connective tissue at the base of each broad ligament, extending from the cervix and vaginal fornix to the side wall of the pelvis. They stabilize the cervix laterally.

The uterosacral ligaments extend from the cervix to the fascia over piriformis, passing on either side of the rectum. They keep the cervix pulled back against the forward pull from the round ligament.

The pubovesical ligaments extend from the cervix and bladder to the pubis laterally.

The parametrium is the tissue lying between the two peritoneal layers of the broad ligament. It contains the uterine and ovarian vessels and lymphatics, the round ligament, and the suspensory ligament of the ovary.

Vessels of the uterus

The uterine artery, a branch of the internal iliac artery, runs in the broad ligament. It anastomoses with branches of the ovarian artery.

Veins run in the broad ligament, to drain eventually into the internal iliac vein.

Ovary

This is an ovoid organ that lies in the ovarian fossa in the angle between the internal and external iliac vessels and closely related to the obturator nerve. It produces the ovum and sex hormones.

The ovary is attached to the posterior leaf of the broad ligament by a double fold of peritoneum, the mesovarium. It is attached to the uterus by the suspensory ligament of the ovary, which runs between the two layers of the broad ligament and is continuous with the round ligament, both being remnants of the gubernaculum.

Blood supply is from the ovarian artery, a branch of the abdominal aorta. It runs in the broad ligament and gives branches to the uterus and uterine tubes. It anastomoses with the uterine artery.

Vagina

This is continuous with the cervix at the external os and opens into the perineum at the vaginal orifice (see Fig. 5.16). The vaginal fornix surrounds the part of the cervix that projects into the vagina. The posterior part of the vaginal fornix is deepest and related to the rectouterine pouch of Douglas. Anteriorly, the vagina is related to the cervix and is separated from the bladder by loose connective tissue.

The upper part of the vagina is supplied by the uterine artery and vaginal branches of the internal iliac, internal pudendal, inferior vesical, and middle rectal arteries. Veins drain into the uterine and vaginal plexuses.

Vessels of the pelvis

The pelvic walls and cavity are supplied by the internal iliac arteries and drain into the internal iliac veins.

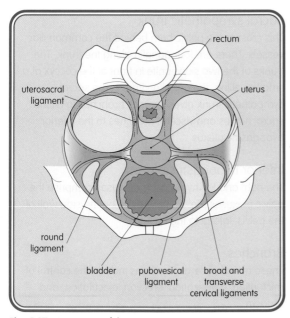

Fig. 5.17 Ligaments of the uterus.

Internal iliac artery

The common iliac artery bifurcates at the pelvic brim opposite the sacroiliac joint into the internal and external iliac arteries (Fig. 5.18). The internal iliac artery passes inferiorly and branches into anterior and posterior divisions. The external iliac artery is concerned mainly with the blood supply to the lower limb.

Internal iliac vein

This commences at the greater sciatic notch by the confluence of the gluteal veins and others that accompany branches of the internal iliac arteries. It passes superiorly and out of the pelvis, lying posterior to the artery on the medial surface of psoas major. Here it joins the external iliac vein to form the common iliac vein.

Tributaries include:
- Veins corresponding to the arteries.
- The uterine and vesicoprostatic venous plexuses.
- The rectal venous plexuses.
- The lateral sacral veins (it communicates with the vertebral venous plexus via these veins).

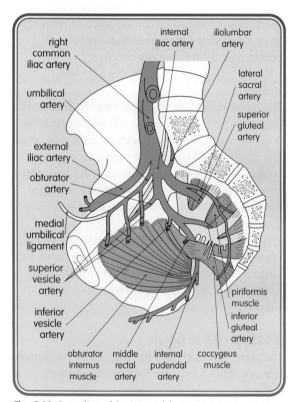

Fig. 5.18 Branches of the internal iliac artery.

Labels (clockwise):
right common iliac artery — internal iliac artery — iliolumbar artery — lateral sacral artery — superior gluteal artery — piriformis muscle — inferior gluteal artery — coccygeus muscle — internal pudendal artery — middle rectal artery — obturator internus muscle — inferior vesicle artery — superior vesicle artery — medial umbilical ligament — obturator artery — external iliac artery — umbilical artery

Nerves of the pelvis
Obturator nerve

This supplies the adductor compartment of the thigh by piercing the medial border of psoas and passing along the side of the pelvis to the obturator foramen.

The ovary is closely related to the obturator nerve—disease of the ovary may cause referred pain to the medial aspect of the thigh and knee.

Sacral plexus

This is formed by the anterior rami of L4 and L5 spinal nerves (the lumbosacral trunk) and the anterior rami of S1–S4 spinal nerves (Fig. 5.19). The plexus lies on the piriformis muscle and is covered by the pelvic fascia. The lateral sacral arteries and veins lie anterior to the plexus. The sacral nerves and the lumbosacral trunk give off branches and then divide into the anterior and posterior divisions.

Sacral sympathetic trunk

This crosses the pelvic brim behind the common iliac vessels. There are four ganglia along the trunk. The trunks of the two sides unite in front of the coccyx at a small swelling, the ganglion impar. The sacral sympathetic trunk gives somatic branches to all the sacral nerves and visceral branches to the inferior hypogastric plexus.

Inferior hypogastric plexus

The right and left hypogastric plexuses comprise the pelvic plexuses (Fig. 5.20). They lie on the side wall of the pelvis, lateral to the rectum.

Branches

These are all visceral. Functions include the control of micturition, defaecation, erection, ejaculation, and orgasm.

Lymphatic drainage of the pelvis

This is summarized in Fig. 5.21.

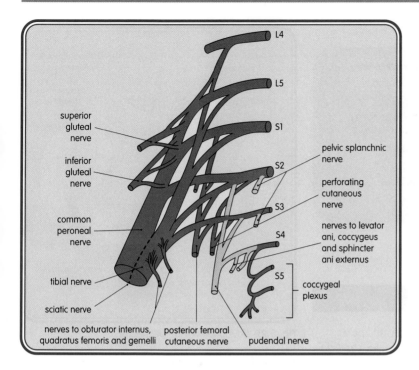

Fig. 5.19 Sacral plexus.

L4

L5

S1

S2

S3

S4

S5

superior gluteal nerve

inferior gluteal nerve

common peroneal nerve

tibial nerve

sciatic nerve

nerves to obturator internus, quadratus femoris and gemelli

posterior femoral cutaneous nerve

pudendal nerve

pelvic splanchnic nerve

perforating cutaneous nerve

nerves to levator ani, coccygeus and sphincter ani externus

coccygeal plexus

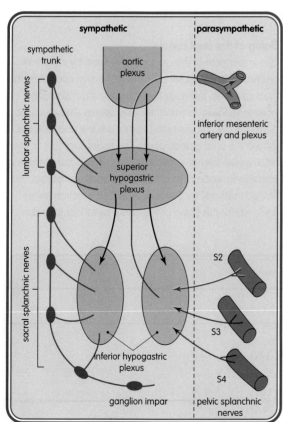

sympathetic

parasympathetic

sympathetic trunk

lumbar splanchnic nerves

sacral splanchnic nerves

aortic plexus

superior hypogastric plexus

inferior hypogastric plexus

ganglion impar

inferior mesenteric artery and plexus

S2

S3

S4

pelvic splanchnic nerves

Fig. 5.20 Autonomic plexuses in the pelvis. (Adapted from *Anatomy as a Basis for Clinical Medicine*, by E.C.B. Hall-Craggs. Courtesy of Williams & Wilkins.)

Lymphatic drainage of the pelvis	
Structure	Lymphatic drainage
anal canal	superficial inguinal nodes
bladder	internal and external iliac nodes
ovary	aortic nodes
rectum	inferior mesenteric nodes internal iliac nodes pararectal nodes preaortic nodes
urethra	internal iliac nodes superficial inguinal nodes
uterus and uterine tubes	external iliac nodes internal iliac nodes sacral nodes
vagina	internal and external iliac nodes superficial inguinal nodes

Fig. 5.21 Lymphatic drainage of the pelvis.

● **Discuss the anatomy of the rectum and bladder.**

● **Describe the anatomy of the structures making up the male and female reproductive tracts.**

● **Outline the vessels and nerves of the pelvis.**

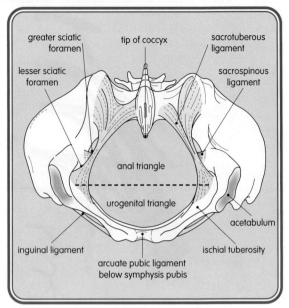

Fig. 5.22 Boundaries of the perineum.

THE PERINEUM

This is the region of the trunk lying below the pelvic diaphragm. It is bounded by the pelvic outlet. Fig. 5.22 illustrates the boundaries of the perineum.

The perineum may be divided into an anterior urogenital triangle and a posterior anal triangle.

Anal triangle

This contains the two ischiorectal fossae separated by the anal canal, the anococcygeal ligament, and the perineal body. Muscles of the anal triangle are outlined in Fig. 5.23.

Anal canal

This commences at the anorectal junction where the rectum passes through the puborectalis muscle. It extends for about 4 cm and ends at the anus.

Lining of the anal canal

The upper part of the anal canal is lined by columnar epithelium with goblet cells that is thrown into folds, the anal columns. Inferiorly these columns are linked by horizontal folds, forming the anal valves. The recesses between the columns and valves are the anal sinuses where the anal glands open. The lower margins of the anal valves form the pectinate line. Below this there is a transitional zone of stratified squamous epithelium, limited inferiorly by the anocutaneous junction (white line), where the lining of the canal becomes true skin.

Muscles of the anal triangle			
Name of muscle (nerve supply)	Origin	Insertion	Action
external anal sphincter—subcutaneous part	encircles anal canal, no bony attachments		voluntary sphincter of anal canal and closes anus
external anal sphincter—superficial part (inferior rectal nerve and perineal branch of fourth sacral nerve)	perineal body	coccyx	
external anal sphincter—deep part	encircles anal canal	coccyx	

Fig. 5.23 Muscles of the anal triangle. (Adapted from *Essential Clinical Anatomy*, 1996, by K.L. Moore. Courtesy of Williams & Wilkins.)

Muscular wall of the anal canal

This surrounds the mucous membrane and is composed of the internal and external anal sphincters (Fig. 5.24).

The internal anal sphincter is a continuation of the circular smooth muscle of the rectum. It surrounds the upper three-quarters of the anal canal and ends at the white line.

The external anal sphincter has subcutaneous, superficial, and deep parts. The muscle is striated and under voluntary control. The external sphincter is supplied by the perineal branch of S4 spinal nerve and the inferior rectal nerve (from the pudendal nerve). Voluntary contraction of the sphincter delays defaecation.

Fig. 5.25 shows the blood supply and lymphatic drainage of the anal canal.

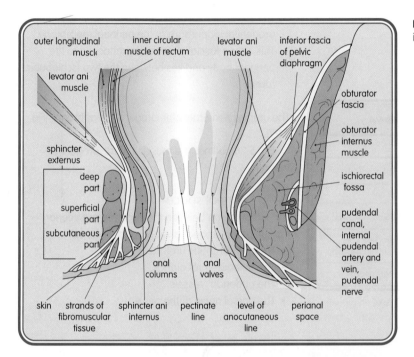

Fig. 5.24 Anal canal and ischiorectal fossa.

Fig. 5.25 Blood supply and lymphatic drainage of the anal canal.

Blood supply and lymphatic drainage of the anal canal	
Arterial supply	**Origin**
superior rectal artery	inferior mesenteric artery
middle rectal artery	internal iliac artery
inferior rectal artery	internal pudendal artery
Venous drainage	**Origin**
internal venous plexus (in submucosa)	superior rectal veins and to inferior mesenteric veins
external venous plexus (outside the muscular coat)	inferior rectal veins drain into internal pudendal veins
muscular coat of the upper part of the canal	middle rectal veins
Lymphatic drainage	**Origin**
upper part of anal canal	nodes alongside the rectum and then to preaortic nodes
lower part of anal canal (above the anocutaneous junction)	internal and common iliac nodes
skin	superficial inguinal nodes

Ischiorectal fossa and pudendal canal

The ischiorectal fossa lies lateral to the anal canal. It is filled with adipose tissue and contains the pudendal canal as well as the the inferior rectal arteries and nerves (see Fig. 5.24). The boundaries of the ischiorectal fossa are detailed in Fig. 5.26.

The pudendal canal lies between the obturator internus and the ischial tuberosity. It contains the internal pudendal vessels and the pudendal nerve, which are conducted from the lesser sciatic foramen to the deep perineal pouch.

Boundaries of the ischiorectal fossa	
Boundary	**Components**
base	skin over anal region of perineum
medial wall	anal canal and levator ani
lateral wall	ischial tuberosity and obturator internus
apex	where levator ani is attached to its tendinous origins over obturator fascia
anterior extension	superior to deep perineal pouch

Fig. 5.26 Boundaries of the ischiorectal fossa.

The male urogenital triangle

The urogenital diaphragm lies below the anterior part of the pelvic floor. It has a layer of striated muscle lying between two fascial layers.

- The deep fascial layer is the superior fascia of the urogenital diaphragm. It blends with the perineal body and the perineal membrane posteriorly.
- The muscle layer consists of the deep transverse perineal muscle and the sphincter urethrae.
- The superficial fascial layer is the inferior fascia of the urogenital diaphragm or the perineal membrane. This strong fascial sheet is also attached to the perineal body and lies between the two ischiopubic rami.

The urethra penetrates the urogenital diaphragm (Fig. 5.27).

Fig. 5.28 outlines the muscles of the urogenital triangle.

Deep perineal space

This is the region beween the superior and inferior fasciae of the urogenital diaphragm. It contains:

- The membranous urethra.
- The bulbourethral glands.
- The pudendal vessels.
- The dorsal nerve of the penis.

Fig. 5.27 Coronal section of the male perineum.

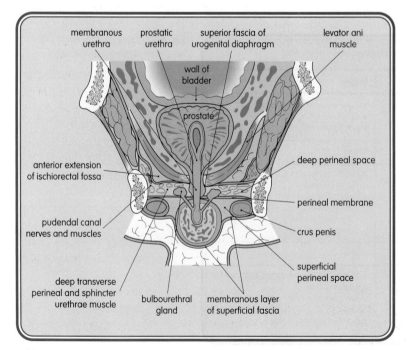

Muscles of the urogenital triangle			
Name of muscle (nerve supply)	**Origin**	**Insertion**	**Action**
superficial transverse perineal muscle (perineal branch of pudendal nerve)	ischial tuberosity	perineal body	fixes perineal body
bulbospongiosus (perineal branch of pudendal nerve)	perineal body and median raphe in male, perineal body in female	fascia of bulb of penis and corpora spongiosum and cavernosum in male, fascia of bulbs of vestibule in female	in male, empties urethra after micturition and ejaculation, and assists in erection of penis; in female, sphincter of vagina and assists in erection of clitoris
ischiocavernosus (perineal branch of pudendal nerve)	ischial tuberosity and ischial ramus in male and female	fascia covering corpus cavernosum	erection of penis or clitoris
deep transverse perineal muscle (perineal branch of pudendal nerve)	ramus of ischium	perineal body	fixes perineal body
sphincter urethrae (perineal branch of pudendal nerve)	pubic arch	surrounds urethra	voluntary sphincter of urethra

Fig. 5.28 Muscles of the urogenital triangle. (Adapted from *Essential Clinical Anatomy*, 1996, by K.L. Moore. Courtesy of Williams & Wilkins.)

The bulbourethral glands are two small glands lying on either side of the membranous urethra (see Fig. 5.26). Their ducts pierce the perineal membrane to enter the spongy part of the urethra. Secretions contribute to the seminal fluid.

Superficial perineal space

This consists of thick areolar tissue. It is attached to the perineal membrane, the ischiopubic rami, and over the thigh where it fuses with the fascia lata. It surrounds the scrotum and the the penis and becomes continuous with the superficial fascia of the anterior abdominal wall.

The male external genitalia

These consist of the penis and the scrotum.

Penis

The penis is suspended from the symphysis pubis. It consists of the root, the shaft, and the glans (Fig. 5.29).

The root is made up of three masses of erectile tissue: the bulb of the penis and the right and left crura. The bulb and crura are partially surrounded by the bulbospongiosus and ischiocavernosus muscles. The

superficial transverse perineal muscle is also closely related to these.

The crura become the corpora cavernosa; the bulb becomes the corpus spongiosum. The urethra passes into the erectile tissue of the bulb and continues in the corpus spongiosum to the external urethral orifice.

The distal end of the corpus spongiosum expands to form the glans penis. The shaft is surrounded by thin loose skin. At the proximal part of the glans penis the skin is reflected upon itself to form the prepuce or foreskin, which covers the glans. The prepuce is attached to the ventral surface of the glans by a fold of skin, the frenulum of the prepuce, which contains a small artery.

The crura and corpora cavernosa receive blood from the deep arteries of the penis. The bulb and corpus spongiosum are supplied by the artery to the bulb and the dorsal artery. The dorsal artery supplies the skin and superficial layers as well.

These vessels allow rapid distension of the cavernous spaces to produce an erection.

Venous drainage is to the deep and superficial dorsal veins.

Parasympathetic vasodilator and sensory fibres enter the penis via the pudendal nerves and their terminal branches, the dorsal nerves of the penis.

Vessels of the male urogenital triangle

The internal pudendal artery is a branch of the internal iliac artery. Its course, distribution and branches are outlined in Fig. 5.30.

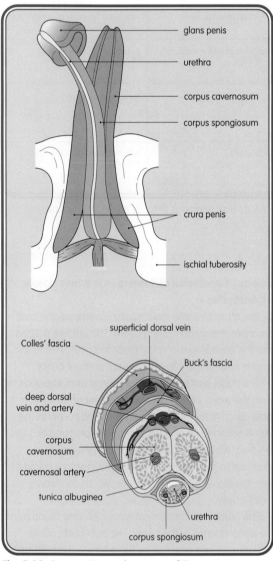

Fig. 5.29 Composition and structure of the penis.

The internal pudendal veins are the venae comitantes of the arteries. The deep dorsal vein of the penis drains into the prostatic plexus. The superficial dorsal vein of the penis drains to a superficial pudendal vein and then to the femoral vein.

Lymphatics of the male urogenital triangle

The penis and scrotum drain into the superficial and deep inguinal nodes.

Nerves of the male urogenital triangle

The pudendal nerve (S2–S4) passes with the internal pudendal artery through the lesser sciatic foramen and the pudendal canal, where it gives rise to the inferior rectal nerve. At the posterior border of the perineal membrane the nerve divides into the perineal nerve and the dorsal nerve of the penis:

- The inferior rectal nerve supplies the external anal sphincter and the skin around the anus.
- The perineal nerve passes superficial to the perineal membrane. It supplies the scrotum posteriorly and all the remaining striated muscles of the perineum.
- The dorsal nerve of the penis runs with the dorsal artery of the penis. It passes over the dorsum of the penis lateral to the artery and terminates in the glans.

The female urogenital triangle

This is similar to the male triangle except for the presence of the vagina.

Perineal membrane

The crura of the clitoris are reattached to the ischiopubic rami. The urethra and vagina divide the membrane, which becomes fused with their outer fascial covering.

Vagina

Superiorly, the vagina passes through the pelvic floor surrounded by part of the puborectalis; anteriorly, it is closely related to the urethra; posteriorly, the perineal body separates it from the anal canal; inferiorly, it opens into the vestibule at the introitus. This opening is partially occluded by a thin membrane, the hymen. The latter is usually destroyed during sexual intercourse.

Fig. 5.30 Internal pudendal artery and its structures.

	Internal pudendal artery and its branches	
Vessel	**Source**	**Course and distribution**
internal pudendal artery	anterior dorsum of internal iliac artery	Exits the pelvis via the greater sciatic foramen to enter the pudendal canal. At the anterior end of the canal it enters the deep perineal pouch and continues forward on the deep surface of the perineal membrane. It terminates by dividing into the dorsal and deep arteries of the penis
inferior rectal artery	internal pudendal artery	Crosses the ischiorectal fossa to supply the muscles and skin of the anal canal
perineal branch	internal pudendal artery	Passes to the superficial perennial space to supply its muscles and the scrotum
artery to bulb of penis	internal pudendal artery	Supplies the erectile tissue of the bulb and corpus spongiosum
deep artery of penis	internal pudendal artery	Supplies the anus and corpus cavernosum
dorsal artery of penis	internal pudendal artery	Passes to the dorsum of the penis. It supplies the erectile tissue of the corpus cavernosum and superficial structures
urethral artery	internal pudendal artery	Supplies the urethra

Clitoris

The clitoris consists of two erectile crura attached to the perineal membrane and ischiopubic rami. Anteriorly, the crura become the corpora cavernosa. These are bound together by fascia to form the body of the clitoris. The glans surmounts the body. It is connected to the bulbs of the vestibule by erectile tissue. These lie on either side of the vaginal orifice.

Perineal body

This is a knot of tissue lying between the vagina and anal canal. The superficial and deep transverse perineal muscles, the pubovaginalis, bulbospongiosus, and the superficial part of the external anal sphincter are attached to it.

Vestibule and labia

The labia minora surround the vestibule and enclose the clitoris (Fig. 5.31). The labia majora lie outside the

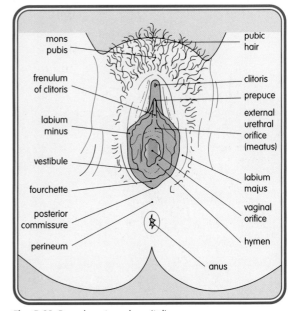

Fig. 5.31 Female external genitalia.

labia minora and fuse with the mons pubis anteriorly. The outer surface of the labia majora is covered with hair, but the inner surface is smooth.

Vessels and nerves of the female urogenital triangle

The internal pudendal artery has a similar course and distribution in the female as in the male, except:

- Posterior labial branches replace scrotal branches.
- The artery to the bulb and vestibule and the dorsal arteries of the clitoris replace the arteries to the penis.

The pudendal nerve is similar in both sexes.

- Discuss the anatomy of the anal canal, ischiorectal fossa, and pudendal canal.
- Outline the structures of the male and female urogenital triangles.
- Describe the male and female external genitalia.

6. The Lower Limb

REGIONS AND COMPONENTS OF THE LOWER LIMB

The lower limb is built for support, locomotion, and the maintenance of equilibrium. Weight is transferred from the rigid bony pelvis, through the acetabulum, to the lower limb. Propulsive movements are transmitted in a similar way but in the opposite direction.

The hip joint is formed by the acetabulum and the head of the femur. It is a very stable joint, with a good range of movement.

The femur articulates with the tibia at the knee joint. Only flexion and extension are possible at this joint. The superior part of the fibula serves for muscle attachment only and does not take part in the formation of the knee joint or in weight bearing.

Both the tibia and the fibula articulate with the tarsal bones to form the ankle joint, where only flexion and extension movements may occur.

The blood supply to the lower limb is from the external iliac artery. This becomes the femoral artery beneath the inguinal ligament and supplies the entire thigh region. Behind the knee the femoral artery becomes the popliteal artery, which supplies the leg and the foot.

The gluteal region is supplied by the superior and inferior gluteal arteries, branches of the internal iliac artery.

The lower limb is innervated by the lumbar and sacral plexuses via the femoral, obturator and sciatic nerves. The gluteal region is also supplied by the superior and inferior gluteal nerves.

SURFACE ANATOMY AND SUPERFICIAL STRUCTURES

Hip and thigh region

The iliac crest and iliac spines should be familiar (pp. 80–81). The greater trochanter of the femur is the widest palpable structure in the hip region.

The large quadriceps muscle makes up the anterior surface of the thigh. It inserts into the patella and, via the patellar tendon, into the tibial tuberosity. The patella is a sesamoid bone in the quadriceps tendon. It may be easily palpated.

The iliotibial tract lies on the lateral surface of the thigh. The gluteus maximus and tensor fasciae latae insert into it. It may be demonstrated with the subject standing on tiptoe.

The hamstrings lie in the posterior compartment of the thigh. They can be demonstrated by attempting to flex the knees against resistance.

Knee region

On the lateral side of the knee the head of the fibula, the lateral part of the tibia, and the lateral condyle of the femur are palpable. Posteriorly the diamond-shaped popliteal fossa is seen when the knees are flexed against resistance.

Leg region

The subcutaneous anteromedial surface of the tibia (shin bone) is easily felt.

Just below the head of the fibula the common peroneal nerve becomes superficial as it runs from the popliteal fossa into the lateral compartment of the leg. It is vulnerable to injury at this point. The peroneal muscles lie laterally on the leg.

The large gastrocnemius and soleus muscles are seen at the back of the leg. These insert into the Achilles tendon.

Ankle

The malleoli are prominences medially and laterally.

Superficial veins

The entire foot drains into the dorsal venous arch, which drains laterally into the small saphenous vein and medially into the great saphenous vein.

Great saphenous vein

The great saphenous vein passes anterior to the medial malleolus and ascends in the subcutaneous tissue on the medial side of the leg and thigh until it reaches the saphenous opening in the fascia lata (Fig. 6.1A). Here it perforates the cribriform fascia covering the opening and joins the femoral vein.

It communicates with the deep veins via perforating veins.

The great saphenous vein is valved, allowing flow of blood in one direction only. Damage to the valves may result in varicose veins.

Tributaries of the great saphenous vein arise from the anterior and medial aspects of the thigh and from the anterior abdominal wall. These include:

- The superficial circumflex iliac vein.
- The superficial epigastric vein.
- The external pudendal vein.

The great saphenous vein is commonly used as a site for cannulation and it may also be used as a graft for a coronary artery bypass operation.

Small saphenous vein

This passes posteriorly to the lateral malleolus and runs superiorly and posteriorly to pierce the deep fascia of the popliteal fossa, where it joins the popliteal vein (Fig. 6.1B). It drains the lateral part of the leg and communicates with the deep veins of the leg via perforating veins.

Lymphatic drainage of the lower limb

Lymphatics from the superficial tissues of the lower limb drain into the superficial inguinal lymph nodes (Fig. 6.2). These lie superficial to the deep fascia around the termination of the saphenous vein. They also receive lymph from the lower part of the perineum, the abdominal wall, and the buttock.

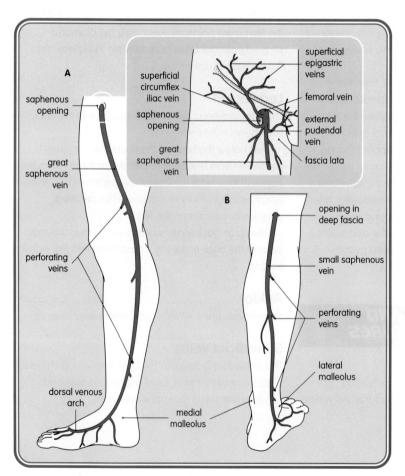

Fig. 6.1 Great (A) and small (B) saphenous veins and their tributaries.

The deep nodes lie alongside the femoral vessels and drain the deep tissues of the lower limb. They communicate with the superficial nodes and their efferent vessels drain into nodes lying alongside the external iliac vessels.

Cutaneous innervation of the lower limb

Figs 6.3 and 6.4 illustrate the dermatomes of the lower limb and its cutaneous innervation, respectively.

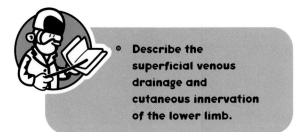

- Describe the superficial venous drainage and cutaneous innervation of the lower limb.

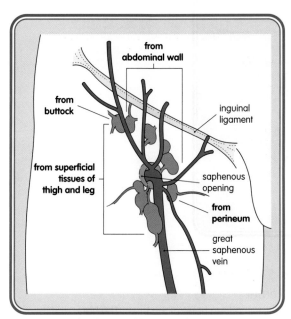

Fig. 6.2 Superficial inguinal lymph nodes.

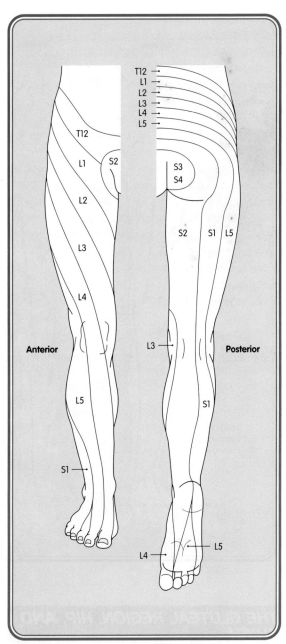

Fig. 6.3 Dermatomes of the lower limb.

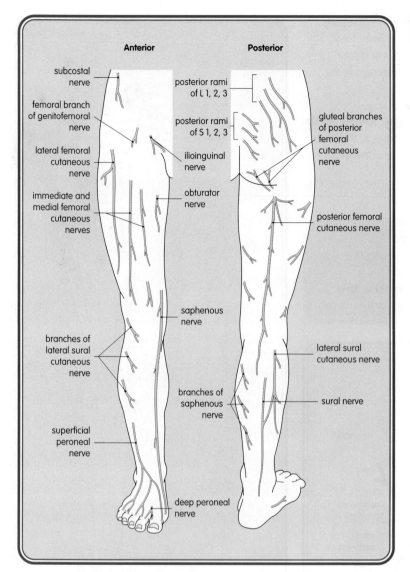

Fig. 6.4 Cutaneous innervation of the lower limb.

Labels (anterior):
- subcostal nerve
- femoral branch of genitofemoral nerve
- lateral femoral cutaneous nerve
- immediate and medial femoral cutaneous nerves
- ilioinguinal nerve
- obturator nerve
- branches of lateral sural cutaneous nerve
- saphenous nerve
- branches of saphenous nerve
- superficial peroneal nerve
- deep peroneal nerve

Labels (posterior):
- posterior rami of L 1, 2, 3
- posterior rami of S 1, 2, 3
- gluteal branches of posterior femoral cutaneous nerve
- posterior femoral cutaneous nerve
- lateral sural cutaneous nerve
- sural nerve

THE GLUTEAL REGION, HIP, AND THIGH

Skeleton of the hip and thigh
Pelvic girdle
This protects the pelvic cavity and supports the body weight. It transmits load to the lower limbs via the sacrum, hip bone, and hip joint (see Chapter 5).

Femur
This is the long bone of the thigh. The bone and its muscle attachments are illustrated in Fig. 6.5.

Fascia lata
This is the deep fascia of the thigh. It lies below the skin and superficial fascia, and encloses the compartments of the thigh.

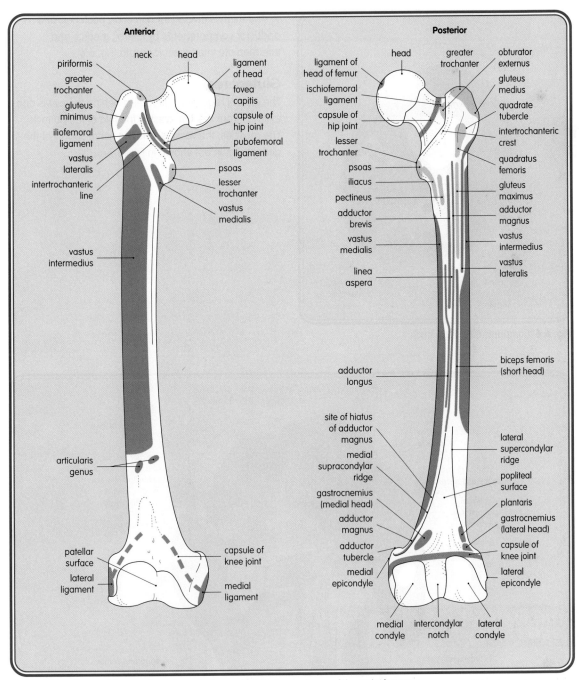

Fig. 6.5 Muscles and ligaments of the anterior and posterior surfaces of the right femur.

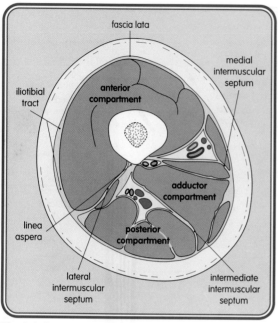

Fig. 6.6 Compartments of the thigh.

The thigh is divided into anterior, posterior, and adductor compartments by lateral, medial, and intermediate intermuscular septa (Fig. 6.6).

Gluteal region

The gluteal region or buttock lies behind the pelvis and extends from the iliac crest to the fold of the buttock. The muscles, the vessels, and the nerve supply of the gluteal region are shown in Figs 6.7–6.10.

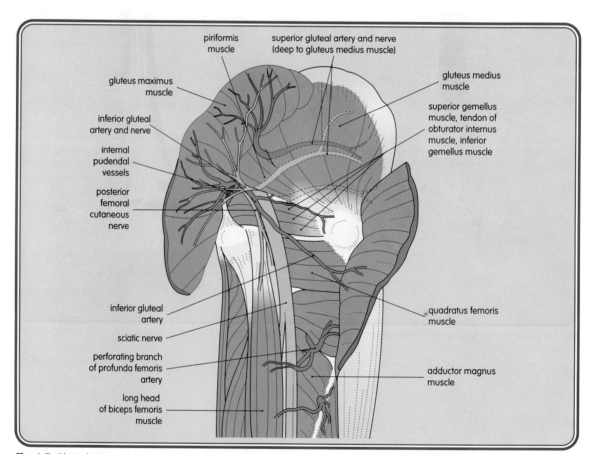

Fig. 6.7 Gluteal region showing the main nerves and vessels.

Muscles of the gluteal region			
Name of muscle (nerve supply)	Origin	Insertion	Action
tensor fasciae latae (superior gluteal nerve)	iliac crest	iliotibial tract	extends knee joint
gluteus maximus (inferior gluteal nerve)	ilium, sacrum, coccyx, and sacrotuberous ligament	iliotibial tract and gluteal tuberosity of femur	extends and laterally rotates thigh at hip joint; extends knee joint
gluteus medius (superior gluteal nerve)	ilium	greater trochanter of femur	abducts thigh at hip joint and tilts pelvis when walking
gluteus minimus (superior gluteal nerve)	ilium	greater trochanter of femur	as gluteus medius and medially rotates thigh
piriformis (S1, S2 nerves)	anterior surface of sacrum	greater trochanter of femur	all these muscles rotate thigh laterally at hip joint
obturator internus (sacral plexus)	inner surface of obturator membrane	greater trochanter of femur	
gemellus inferior (sacral plexus)	ischial tuberosity	greater trochanter of femur	
gemellus superior (sacral plexus)	ischial spine	greater trochanter of femur	
quadratus femoris (sacral plexus)	ischial spine	quadrate tubercle on femur	

Fig. 6.8 Muscles of the gluteal region.

The buttock is a common site for intramuscular injections. The sciatic nerve is at risk of damage unless injections are given in the upper outer quadrant.

Arteries of the gluteal region	
Artery	Course and distribution
internal pudendal	passes through the greater sciatic foramen to enter the gluteal region, then passes into the perineum via the lesser sciatic foramen; supplies the muscles of the pelvic region and the external genitalia
superior gluteal	enters the gluteal region through the greater sciatic foramen; supplies gluteus maximus, medius and minimus, and tensor fasciae latae
inferior gluteal	passes through the greater sciatic foramen to enter the gluteal region; supplies gluteus maximus, obturator internus, and quadratus femoris

Fig. 6.9 Arteries of the gluteal region.

Nerves of the gluteal region	
Nerve (origin)	**Course and distribution**
inferior gluteal (anterior rami of L5–S2)	leaves pelvis through greater sciatic foramen, and supplies gluteus maximus
superior gluteal (anterior rami of L4–S1)	leaves pelvis through greater sciatic foramen and passes between gluteus medius and minimus to supply these muscles and tensor fasciae latae
nerve to quadratus femoris (anterior rami of L4, L5, and S1)	leaves pelvis through greater sciatic foramen to supply the hip joint, inferior gemellus, and quadratus femoris
nerve to obturator internus (anterior rami of L5, S1, and S2)	enters gluteal region through greater sciatic foramen, descends posterior to ischial spine, enters lesser sciatic foramen, and passes to obturator internus to supply it and superior gemellus
posterior femoral cutaneous (sacral plexus—S1–S3)	leaves pelvis through greater sciatic foramen, runs deep to gluteus maximus, and emerges from its inferior border to supply skin of buttock and then surface skin over posterior of thigh and calf
pudenal (anterior rami of S2–S4)	enters gluteal region through greater sciatic foramen, descends posterior to sacrospinous ligament, enters perineum through lesser sciatic foramen, and supplies the latter
sciatic (sacral plexus—L4–S3)	leaves pelvis through greater sciatic foramen, to enter gluteal region—it has no motor branches in the gluteal region

Fig. 6.10 Nerves of the gluteal region.

Muscles of the anterior compartment of the thigh			
Name of muscle (nerve supply)	**Origin**	**Insertion**	**Action**
quadriceps femoris—rectus femoris; vastus lateralis, medialis, and intermedius (femoral nerve)	ilium and upper part of femur	quadriceps tendon into patella then patellar tendon onto tibia	extends leg at knee joint
sartorius (femoral nerve)	anterior superior iliac spine	shaft of tibia	flexes, abducts, and laterally rotates thigh at hip joint; flexes and medially rotates leg at knee joint
psoas major (lumbar plexus)	T12 body, transverse processes, bodies, and intervertebral discs L1–L5	lesser tronchanter of femur	flexes thigh or trunk
iliacus (femoral nerve)	iliac fossa of hip bone	lesser trochanter of femur	flexes thigh on trunk
pectineus (femoral nerve)	superior ramus of pubis	upper shaft of femur	flexes and adducts thigh at hip joint

Fig. 6.11 Muscles of the anterior compartment of the thigh.

Anterior compartment of the thigh

This is bound anterolaterally by the fascia lata. The medial intermuscular septum separates it from the adductor compartment, and the lateral intermuscular septum separates the extensor compartment from the flexor compartment.

The muscles of the anterior compartment are described in Fig. 6.11.

Femoral triangle

This contains the femoral artery, vein, and nerve (Fig. 6.12). These all lie superficially just beneath the skin, superficial fascia, and fascia lata.

The femoral artery and vein and the femoral canal are enclosed by the femoral sheath, a thickening derived from the transversalis and iliac fasciae. The femoral nerve is separated from the femoral sheath by the iliopectineal fascia.

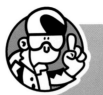

The arrangement of the femoral vessels and nerve as they pass under the inguinal ligament can be remembered as 'NAVY' (nerve, artery, vein, Y-fronts!).

Fig. 6.12 Femoral triangle and its contents.

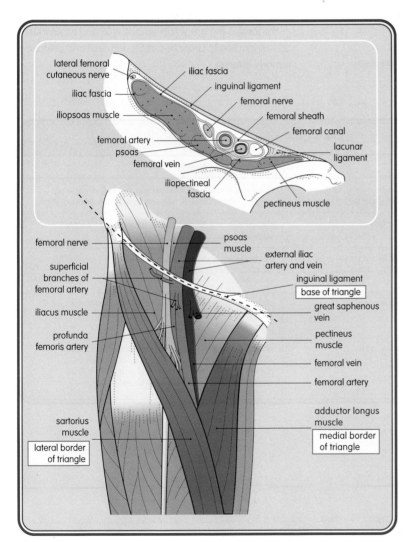

Femoral canal

This contains efferent lymphatics passing from the deep inguinal nodes to the abdomen (see Fig. 6.12). It provides space for expansion of the femoral vein during times of increased venous return from the lower limb. Its boundaries are the medial part of the inguinal ligament, the lacunar ligament, the femoral vein, and pectineus.

Adductor canal

At the apex of the femoral triangle the femoral vessels disappear beneath sartorius and follow the muscle to the medial aspect of the thigh in a channel, the adductor canal.

It is bounded laterally by the vastus medialis and posteromedially by the adductor longus and adductor magnus.

Vessels of the thigh

Fig. 6.13 outlines the arterial supply of the thigh.

Cruciate anastomosis

This provides an alternative circulation should the femoral artery be obstructed. It is made up of:

- The inferior gluteal branch of the internal iliac artery.
- The medial and lateral circumflex femoral arteries.
- The first perforating artery.

All the perforating arteries anastomose with each other and with the muscular branches of the popliteal artery. In this way the internal iliac artery and the popliteal artery are linked.

Femoral vein

This lies posterior to the artery in the adductor canal. Below the inguinal ligament the vein lies medial to the artery in the femoral sheath. It passes behind the inguinal ligament to become the external iliac vein.

It receives the great saphenous vein and tributaries corresponding to branches of the femoral and profunda femoris arteries.

Arterial supply to the thigh		
Artery	**Origin**	**Course and distribution**
femoral	continuation of external iliac artery distal to inguinal ligament	descends through femoral triangle and enters adductor canal; supplies anterior and anteromedial surfaces of thigh
profunda femoris	femoral artery	passes inferiorly, deep to adductor longus, to supply posterior compartment of thigh
lateral circumflex femoral	profunda femoris; may arise from femoral artery	passes laterally deep to sartorius and rectus femoris to supply anterior part of gluteal region, and femur and knee joint
medial circumflex femoral	profunda femoris	passes medially and posteriorly between pectineus and iliopsoas, and enters gluteal region; supplies head and neck of femur
obturator	internal iliac artery	passes through obturator foramen and enters medial compartment of thigh; supplies obturator externus, pectineus, adductors of thigh, and gracilis—muscles attached to ischial tuberosity and head of femur

Fig. 6.13 Arterial supply to the thigh.

Nerves of the thigh
The nerves of the thigh region are outlined in Fig. 6.14.

Adductor compartment of the thigh
The muscles of the adductor compartment are outlined in Fig. 6.15. They are all supplied by the obturator nerve except for the part of the adductor magnus muscle that

belongs to the posterior compartment, which is supplied by the sciatic nerve (see Fig. 6.14).

The perforating branches of the profunda femoris artery and the muscular branches of the femoral artery provide the majority of the blood supply to the adductor compartment. The obturator artery also contributes proximally to the blood supply of this region.

Fig. 6.14 Nerves of the thigh.

Nerves of the thigh	
Nerve (origin)	**Course and distribution**
ilioinguinal (lumbar plexus—L1)	supplies skin over femoral triangle
genitofemoral (lumbar plexus—L1–L2)	descends on anterior surface of psoas major and divides into genital and femoral branches: femoral branch supplies skin over femoral triangle; genital branch supplies scrotum or labia majora
lateral femoral cutaneous (lumbar plexus—L2–L3)	passes deep to inguinal ligament, 2–3 cm medial to anterior superior iliac spine; supplies skin on anterior and lateral aspects of thigh
medial and intermediate femoral cutaneous (femoral nerve)	arise in femoral triangle and pierce fascia lata of thigh; supply skin on medial and anterior aspect of thigh
posterior femoral cutaneous (sacral plexus—S2–S3)	passes through greater sciatic foramen; supplies skin over posterior aspect of thigh and the buttock
femoral (lumbar plexus—L2–L4)	passes deep to inguinal ligament; supplies anterior thigh muscles, hip and knee joints, and skin on anteromedial side of thigh
obturator (lumbar plexus—L2–L4)	enters thigh through obturator foramen and divides: anterior branch supplies adductor longus, adductor brevis, gracilis, and pectineus; posterior branch supplies obturator externus and adductor magnus
sciatic (sacral plexus—L4–S3)	enters gluteal region through greater sciatic foramen, descends along posterior aspect of thigh, and divides proximal to knee into tibial and common peroneal nerves; innervates hamstrings by its tibial division (except for short head of biceps femoris) and has articular branches to hip and knee joints

Muscles of the adductor compartment of the thigh			
Name of muscle (nerve supply)	**Origin**	**Insertion**	**Action**
adductor brevis (obturator nerve)	inferior ramus of pubis	posterior surface of femur	adducts thigh at hip joint
adductor longus (obturator nerve)	body of pubis	posterior surface of femur	adducts thigh at hip joint
adductor magnus (adductor part—obturator nerve; hamstring part—sciatic nerve)	ischiopubic ramus	posterior surface of femur, adductor tubercle of femur	adducts thigh at hip joint; hamstring part extends thigh at hip joint
gracilis (obturator nerve)	ischiopubic ramus	upper part of tibia	adducts thigh at hip joint
obturator externus (obturator nerve)	outer surface of obturator membrane	greater trochanter of femur	lateral rotation of thigh at hip joint

Fig. 6.15 Muscles of the adductor compartment of the thigh.

Posterior compartment of the thigh

The muscles of the posterior compartment are outlined in Fig. 6.16 and illustrated in Fig. 6.17. They are all supplied by the sciatic nerve (see Fig. 6.14).

Blood supply to the posterior compartment is mainly from the perforating branches of the profunda femoris, with a small contribution from the inferior gluteal artery.

Hip joint

This is a ball-and-socket synovial joint comprising articulation between the acetabulum and the head of the femur. It is a very stable joint (unlike the shoulder joint) and exhibits a high degree of mobility.

Stability is mainly achieved from the close fit between the femoral head and the acetabulum. Great mobility is achieved because the femoral neck is much narrower than the diameter of the head so that considerable movement may occur in all directions before the neck impinges on the acetabular labrum.

The articular surface of the acetabulum is covered by hyaline cartilage. The peripheral edge of this surface is deepened by a rim of fibrocartilage, the acetabular labrum. The labrum thus contributes further to joint stability. The labrum continues across the acetabular notch as the transverse ligament.

The articular surface of the head of the femur is also covered by hyaline cartilage. The non-articular convexity of the head is excavated into a pit (fovea) for attachment of the ligament of the head of the femur.

The capsule is attached around the labrum and transverse ligament and the neck of the femur. Over the femoral neck the capsule is thrown into folds called retinacula. It is loose and strong. A synovial membrane lines its internal surface.

The capsule is reinforced by three strong ligaments that extend from the pelvic bone to the femur:
- The pubofemoral ligament.
- The ischiofemoral ligament.
- The iliofemoral ligament.

Blood supply is from branches of the following:
- The medial circumflex femoral artery.
- The superior gluteal artery.
- The inferior gluteal artery.
- The obturator artery.

Nerve supply comprises the following:
- The femoral nerve.
- The sciatic nerve.
- The obturator nerve.

Muscles of the posterior compartment of the thigh			
Name of muscle (nerve supply)	Origin	Insertion	Action
biceps femoris (sciatic neve)	ischial tuberosity linea aspera–femur	head of fibula	all the muscles flex the leg at the knee joint and extend the thigh at the hip joint
semitendinosus (sciatic nerve)	ischial tuberosity	upper part of shaft of tibia	
semimembranosus (sciatic nerve)	ischial tuberosity	medial condyle of tibia, forms oblique popliteal ligament	

Fig. 6.16 Muscles of the posterior compartment of the thigh.

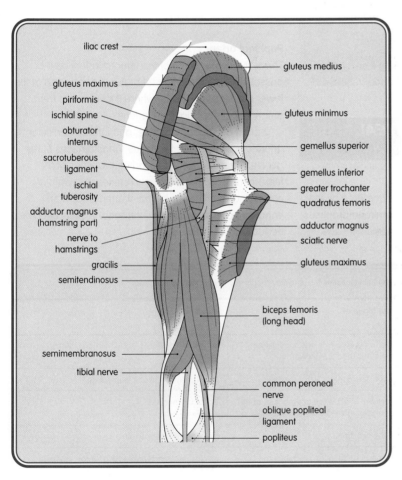

Fig. 6.17 Structure of the posterior aspect of the right thigh. The short head of biceps femoris has been removed to show deeper structures.

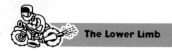
Movements of the hip joint

Any movement of the shaft of the femur is accompanied by a different movement of the neck and head (Fig. 6.18).

- Outline the skeleton of the hip and thigh region.
- Discuss the muscles of the anterior, posterior, and adductor compartments of the thigh.
- List the vessels and nerves of the lower limb.
- Describe the femoral triangle and its contents.

THE KNEE AND POPLITEAL FOSSA

Popliteal fossa

The diamond-shaped popliteal fossa is bordered by the biceps femoris, semitendinosus, and semimembranosus muscles superiorly and by the gastrocnemius muscle inferiorly (Fig. 6.19). It is roofed by the deep fascia, which is pierced by the small saphenous vein and lymphatics. The floor is formed by the body of the femur, the oblique popliteal ligament, and the popliteus muscle.

Contents of the popliteal fossa

Popliteus muscle

This has the following characteristics:

- Origin—a pit just below the lateral epicondyle of the femur and the lateral meniscus of the knee joint. It is intracapsular.
- Insertion—popliteal surface of the tibia.
- Nerve supply—tibial nerve.
- Action—unlocks the knee and draws the lateral meniscus posteriorly.

Popliteal artery

This is the continuation of the femoral artery as it passes through the adductor hiatus. It terminates at the lower border of popliteus, where it divides into the anterior and posterior tibial arteries.

It gives off superior, middle, and inferior genicular arteries and muscular branches. Anastomoses of the genicular vessels with descending branches of the femoral and profunda femoris arteries and with ascending branches of the tibial arteries form an important collateral supply if the main vessels become occluded.

Movements of the hip joint and the muscles responsible for these movements		
Movement of the thigh on the trunk	**Movement at the hip joint**	**Muscles**
flexion	rotation around a transverse axis passing through both acetabula moving the thigh forwards	psoas major, iliacus, rectus femoris, tensor fasciae latae
extension	as above (opposite direction)	gluteus maximus and hamstrings
adduction	rotation of the femoral head in the acetabulum about an anteroposterior axis moving the thigh medially	adductor muscles
abduction	as above (opposite direction)	gluteus medius and minimus
rotation	rotation of the femoral head in the acetabulum about a vertical axis—which also passes through the knee	medial rotation: tensor fasciae latae, gluteus medius and minimus; lateral rotation: the obturator muscles, piriformis, quadratus femoris

Fig. 6.18 Movements of the hip joint and the muscles responsible for these movements.

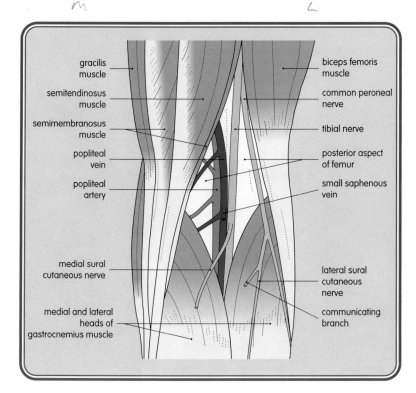

Fig. 6.19 Popliteal fossa and its contents.

Labels on figure:
- gracilis muscle
- semitendinosus muscle
- semimembranosus muscle
- popliteal vein
- popliteal artery
- medial sural cutaneous nerve
- medial and lateral heads of gastrocnemius muscle
- biceps femoris muscle
- common peroneal nerve
- tibial nerve
- posterior aspect of femur
- small saphenous vein
- lateral sural cutaneous nerve
- communicating branch

Popliteal vein

This passes up the popliteal fossa medial to and then superficial to the artery before entering the adductor hiatus. It receives the small saphenous vein together with veins corresponding to the arterial branches.

Common peroneal nerve

This lies beneath the biceps femoris in the popliteal fossa until it reaches the head of the fibula. Branches in the popliteal fossa include:

- The lateral sural nerve, which supplies the skin of the calf.
- A communicating branch with the medial sural nerve.
- Branches to the knee joint.

Tibial nerve

This bisects the popliteal fossa vertically. Branches in the fossa include:

- Articular branches to the knee.

- Muscular branches to soleus, gastrocnemius, plantaris, and popliteus.
- The medial sural cutaneous nerve, which joins the communicating branch of the lateral sural cutaneous nerve to form the sural nerve. The sural nerve supplies the lateral side of the calf and heel. Cutaneous innervation was discussed earlier.

Skeleton of the knee

The main features of the skeleton around the knee are illustrated in Fig 6.20.

Knee joint

This is an articulation between the femur and the tibia, with the patella articulating with the femur anteriorly. It is a synovial joint.

The articular surfaces are covered by hyaline cartilage and consist of the margins of the femoral condyles, the patella, and the superior surface of the tibial condyles.

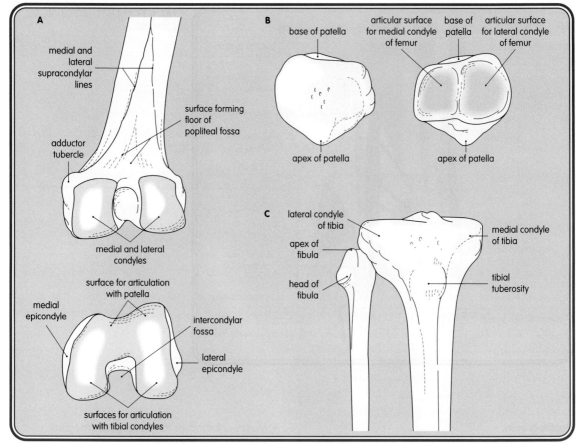

Fig. 6.20 Skeleton of the knee. (A) Posterior and inferior aspects of the lower end of the right femur. (B) Anterior and posterior aspects of the patella. (C) Anterior aspect of the upper end of the right tibia and fibula.

Capsule

The capsule surrounds the articular surfaces but is not complete: it is defective anterosuperiorly, to allow communication between the joint cavity and the suprapatellar bursa, posteroinferiorly, to allow entry of the popliteus tendon, and anteriorly it is replaced by the articular surface of the patella.

The capsule is strengthened anteriorly by the patellar retinacula—expansions of the vastus medialis and lateralis. It is also reinforced by the quadriceps tendon, the patella, and the patella ligament.

Synovial membrane

The synovial membrane lines the capsule (Fig. 6.21). Above the patella it becomes continuous with the lining of the suprapatellar bursa. The cruciate ligaments lie outside the synovial cavity.

Ligaments

Ligaments play a major role in stabilizing the knee joint (Fig. 6.22). The cruciate ligaments keep the articular surfaces applied to each other throughout the range of movement.

Menisci

These are two crescentic plates of fibrocartilage (Fig. 6.23). The horns of the menisci are attached to the intercondylar area of the tibia and at the periphery to the loose coronary ligament of the capsule and to the deep part of the tibial collateral ligament. They increase the congruity of the articular surfaces.

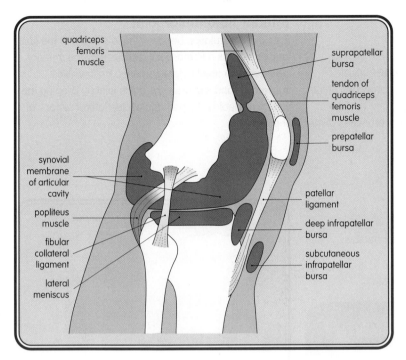

Fig. 6.21 Synovial membrane and its ligaments.

Ligaments of the knee joint	
Ligament	**Attachment**
patellar	the termination of the quadriceps tendon running from the patella to the tibial tuberosity; its tension is controlled by the quadriceps muscle, which stabilizes the joint through its full range of movement
tibial collateral	from the medial femoral condyle to the tibia
fibular collateral	from the lateral femoral condyle to the fibular head
oblique popliteal	expansion of the semi-membranosus tendon, which reinforces the capsule posteriorly
anterior cruciate	from the anterior part of the intercondylar area of the tibia to the medial surface of the lateral femoral condyle
posterior cruciate	from the posterior part of the intercondylar area of the tibia to the lateral surface of the medial femoral condyle

Fig. 6.22 Ligaments of the knee joint.

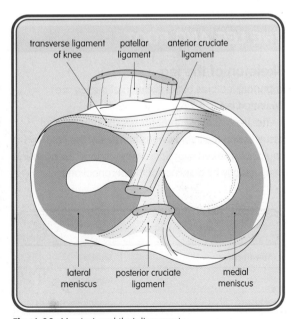

Fig. 6.23 Menisci and their ligaments.

113

Movements at the knee joint

These are outlined in Fig. 6.24.

Blood and nerve supply of the knee joint

Blood supply comes from the genicular branches of the popliteal artery.

Nerve supply comprises the articular branches of the sciatic, femoral, and obturator nerves.

Bursae around the knee joint

These include:

- The suprapatellar bursa.
- The prepatellar bursa.
- The superficial and deep infrapatellar bursae.

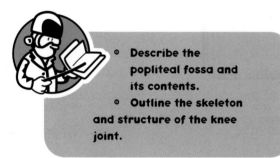

- ◉ **Describe the popliteal fossa and its contents.**
- ◉ **Outline the skeleton and structure of the knee joint.**

THE LEG AND FOOT

Skeleton of the leg

Important features of the skeleton of the leg are illustrated in Fig. 6.25.

The interosseous membrane is a tough band of tissue linking the interosseous borders of the tibia and fibula. It is pierced superiorly by the anterior tibial artery and inferiorly by branches of the peroneal artery.

Movements at the knee joint	
Movement	Muscle
flexion	hamstring
extension	quadriceps femoris
medial and lateral rotation (of the flexed knee)	hamstring

Fig. 6.24 Movements at the knee joint.

Inferior tibiofibular joint

This is an articulation between the lower end of the tibia and fibula. It is a fibrous joint stabilized by the anterior and posterior tibiofibular ligaments. It allows little movement and stabilizes the ankle joint by keeping the lateral malleolus clasped against the lateral surface of the talus.

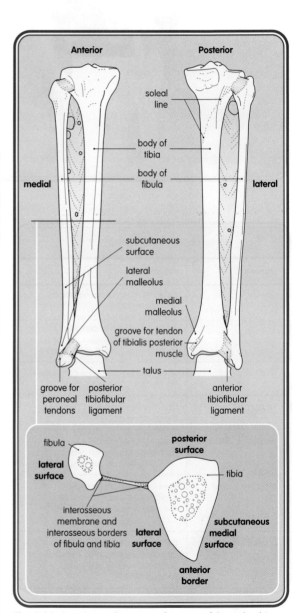

Fig. 6.25 Anterior and posterior features of the right tibia and fibula, and the relationship of the two bones and the interosseous membrane in cross-section.

Compartments of the leg

The leg is divided into anterior, posterior, and lateral compartments (Fig. 6.26). The muscles of the posterior compartment are divided into superficial and deep groups by the transverse crural fascia.

Anterior compartment of the leg

Muscles of the anterior compartment are shown in Figs 6.27 and 6.28.

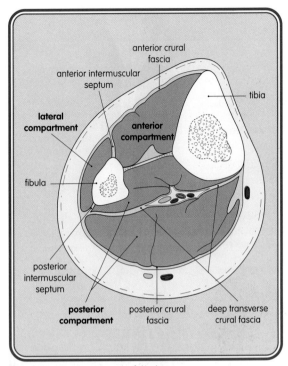

Fig. 6.26 Compartments of the leg.

Muscles of the anterior compartment of the leg			
Name of muscle (nerve supply)	**Origin**	**Insertion**	**Action**
extensor digitorum longus (deep peroneal nerve)	fibula and interosseous membrane	extensor expansion of lateral four toes	extends toes and dorsiflexes foot
extensor hallucis longus (deep peroneal nerve)	fibula and interosseous membrane	base of distal phalanx of great toe	extends big toe, dorsiflexes and inverts foot
peroneus tertius (deep peroneal nerve)	fibula and interosseous membrane	base of 5th metatarsal bone	dorsiflexes and everts foot
tibialis anterior (deep peroneal nerve)	tibia and interosseous membrane	medial cuneiform and base of 1st metatarsal bone	dorsiflexes and inverts foot

Fig. 6.27 Muscles of the anterior compartment of the leg.

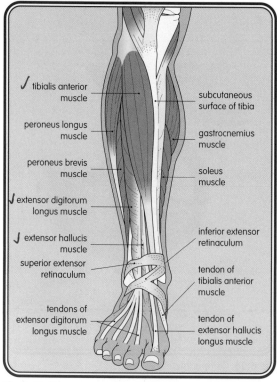

Fig. 6.28 Extensor muscles of the anterior compartment of the leg.

Vessels of the anterior compartment

The anterior tibial artery is the vessel of the anterior compartment (Figs 6.29 and 6.30). It is a terminal branch of the popliteal artery.

Nerves of the anterior compartment

The common peroneal nerve (L4–L5, S1–S2) leaves the popliteal fossa to enter the lateral compartment of the leg by winding around the neck of the fibula (Fig. 6.31). Here it divides into the superficial and deep peroneal nerves.

The common peroneal nerve is vulnerable to injury, e.g. by a car bumper, as it passes around the fibula. Damage results in footdrop.

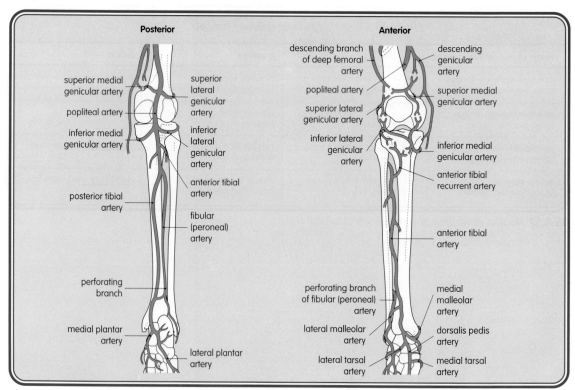

Fig. 6.29 Arterial supply to the posterior and anterior compartments of the leg.

Arterial supply to the leg		
Artery (origin)	**Course**	**Distribution**
popliteal (continuation of femoral artery at adductor hiatus)	passes through popliteal fossa to leg; ends at lower border of popliteus muscle by dividing into anterior and posterior tibial arteries	superior, middle, and inferior genicular arteries to both lateral and medial aspects of knee
anterior tibial (popliteal artery)	passes into anterior compartment through gap in superior part of interosseous membrane and descends on this membrane	anterior compartment of leg
dorsalis pedis (continuation of anterior tibial artery distal to extensor retinaculum)	descends anteromedially to first interosseous space and divides into plantar and arcuate arteries	muscles on dorsum of foot; pierces first dorsal interosseous muscle to contribute to formation of plantar arch
posterior tibial (popliteal artery)	passes through posterior compartment of leg and terminates distal to flexor retinaculum by dividing into medial and lateral plantar arteries	posterior and lateral compartments of leg; nutrient artery passes to tibia, contributes to knee anastomoses
peroneal (posterior tibial artery)	descends in posterior compartment adjacent to posterior intermuscular septum	posterior compartment of leg; perforating branches supply lateral compartment of leg

Fig. 6.30 Arterial supply to the leg.

Fig. 6.31 Nerves of the leg.

Nerves of the leg	
Nerve (origin)	**Course and distribution**
common peroneal (sciatic nerve)	arises at apex of popliteal fossa and follows medial border of biceps femoris and its tendon; passes over posterior aspect of head of fibula and then winds around neck of fibula, deep to peroneus longus, where it divides into deep and superficial peroneal nerves; supplies skin on posterolateral part of leg via its branch —lateral sural cutaneous nerve
deep peroneal (common peroneal nerve)	arises between peroneus longus and neck of fibula; descends on interosseous membrane and enters dorsum of foot; supplies anterior muscles of leg, and skin of first interdigital cleft
saphenous (femoral nerve)	descends with femoral vessels and the great saphenous vein to supply skin on medial side of leg and foot
superficial peroneal (common peroneal nerve)	arises between peroneus longus and neck of fibula and descends in lateral compartment of leg; supplies peroneus longus and brevis and skin on anterior surface of leg and dorsum of foot
sural (usually arises from both tibial and common peroneal nerves)	descends between heads of gastrocnemius and becomes superficial at middle of leg; supplies skin on posterolateral aspects of leg and lateral side of foot
tibial (sciatic nerve)	descends through popliteal fossa and lies on popliteus; then runs inferiorly with posterior tibial vessels and terminates beneath flexor retinaculum by dividing into medial and lateral plantar nerves; supplies posterior muscles of leg and knee joint

Dorsum of the foot

The structures from the anterior compartment pass onto the dorsum of the foot.

The extensor digitorum brevis muscle is the only muscle intrinsic to the dorsum of the foot.

Cutaneous innervation of the dorsum of the foot is from the superficial peroneal nerve, the deep peroneal nerve, the sural nerve, and the saphenous nerve.

Extensor retinacula

The superior and inferior extensor retinacula keep the extensor tendons firmly bound down to the dorsum of the foot (Fig. 6.32). The retinacula are derived from the anterior crural fascia.

The superior band passes from the anterior border of the tibia to the anterior border of the fibula. The inferior band is Y-shaped and runs from the calcaneus to the medial malleolus and plantar fascia.

Nerves and vessels of the dorsum of the foot

The deep peroneal nerve and anterior tibial artery enter the foot beneath the extensor retinacula. The anterior tibial artery continues as the dorsalis pedis artery (see Fig. 6.30).

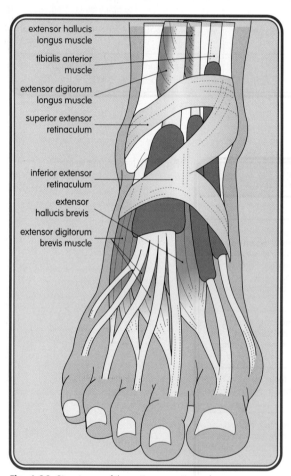

Fig. 6.32 Structures of the extensor retinacula.

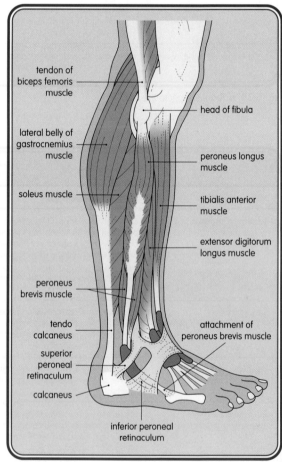

Fig. 6.33 Lateral compartment of the leg and its structures.

Lateral compartment of the leg

The composition of the lateral compartment is shown in Fig. 6.33. Its muscles are outlined in Fig. 6.34.

Posterior compartment of the leg

Fig. 6.35 outlines the muscles of the posterior compartment.

Muscles of the lateral compartment of the leg			
Name of muscle (nerve supply)	**Origin**	**Insertion**	**Action**
peroneus longus (superficial peroneal nerve)	fibula	1st metatarsal and medial cuneiform	plantarflexes and everts the foot
peroneus brevis (superficial peroneal nerve)	fibula	5th metatarsal bone	plantarflexes and everts the foot

Fig. 6.34 Muscles of the lateral compartment of the leg.

Muscles of the posterior compartment of the leg			
Superficial group			
Name of muscle (nerve supply)	**Origin**	**Insertion**	**Action**
plantaris (tibial nerve)	lateral supracondylar ridge of femur	calcaneum	these muscles plantarflex the foot at the ankle joint
soleus (tibial nerve)	tibia and fibula	via tendo calcaneus (Achilles tendon) into calcaneum	
gastrocnemius (tibial nerve)	medial and lateral condyles of femur	via tendo calcaneus (Achilles tendon) into calcaneum	
Deep group			
Name of muscle (nerve supply)	**Origin**	**Insertion**	**Action**
flexor digitorum longus (tibial nerve)	tibia	distal phalanges of lateral four toes	flexes lateral four toes; plantarflexes foot
flexor hallucis longus (tibial nerve)	tibia	distal phalanx of big toe	flexes big toe; plantarflexes foot
tibialis posterior (tibial nerve)	tibia and fibula and interosseous membrane	navicular bone and surrounding bones	plantarflexes and inverts foot

Fig. 6.35 Muscles of the posterior compartment of the leg.

Flexor retinaculum

This runs from the medial malleolus to the calcaneus and plantar fascia (Fig. 6.36). The deep flexor muscles pass beneath the retinaculum surrounded by synovial sheaths together with the tibial nerve and the posterior tibial artery.

Skeleton of the foot

This consists of the tarsal bones, the metatarsal bones, and the phalanges (Fig. 6.37).

The body weight is transferred to the talus and the calcaneus, and then across the remaining tarsal and metatarsal bones. The weight is transferred to the ground at the tuber calcanei and the heads of the metatarsals. The metatarsal bones are composed of a base proximally, a body, and a distal head. The first digit (the hallux) has two phalanges; the others have three (proximal, middle, and distal).

Ankle joint

This is the articulation between the upper surface of the talus and the lower end of the tibia and fibula, including the medial and lateral malleoli.

It is a synovial joint and allows only flexion and extension. Dorsiflexion (extension) involves tibialis anterior, extensor digitorum longus, and extensor hallucis longus. Plantarflexion (flexion) involves gastrocnemius, soleus, and tibialis posterior.

The joint is surrounded by a capsule that is lax anteroposteriorly and reinforced by strong medial and lateral ligaments. The medial (deltoid) ligament runs from the medial malleolus to the tuberosity of the navicular bone, the sustentaculum tali, and the medial tubercle of the talus. The lateral ligament arises from the lateral malleolus and is inserted into the neck of the talus, the calcaneus, and the lateral tubercle of the talus.

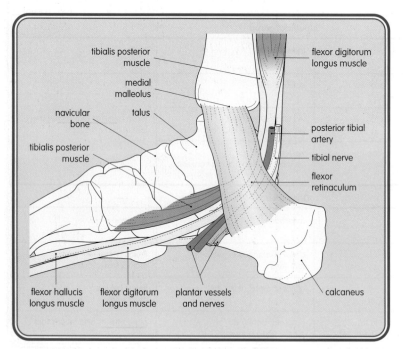

Fig. 6.36 Flexor retinaculum.

The ankle is the most frequently injured joint in the body. The lateral ligament is slightly weaker than the medial ligament and is therefore usually damaged. Severe damage to the ligament results in an unstable joint.

Blood supply is from the anterior and posterior tibial arteries.

Nerve supply is from the tibial and deep peroneal nerves.

Sole of the foot

The sole bears the weight of the body. The skin is thick and hairless. Fibrous septa divide the subcutaneous fat into small loculi and anchor the skin to the deep fascia or plantar aponeurosis (Fig. 6.38)

The plantar aponeurosis extends from the calcaneal tuberosity to the base of the toes. It is very strong and protects the underlying muscles, vessels, and nerves. It is perforated by the cutaneous nerves supplying the sole of the foot.

The muscles of the sole of the foot are in four layers.

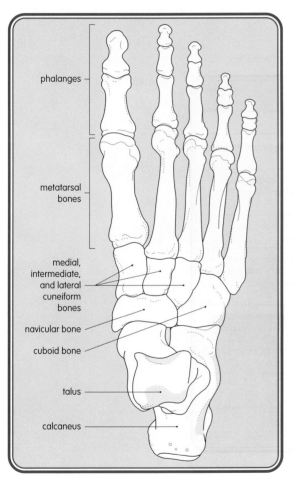

phalanges

metatarsal bones

medial, intermediate, and lateral cuneiform bones

navicular bone

cuboid bone

talus

calcaneus

Fig. 6.37 Skeleton of the foot.

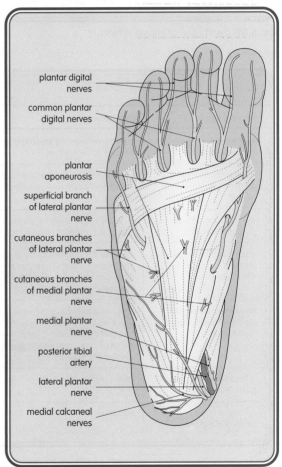

plantar digital nerves

common plantar digital nerves

plantar aponeurosis

superficial branch of lateral plantar nerve

cutaneous branches of lateral plantar nerve

cutaneous branches of medial plantar nerve

medial plantar nerve

posterior tibial artery

lateral plantar nerve

medial calcaneal nerves

Fig. 6.38 Plantar fascia and cutaneous innervation of the sole of the foot.

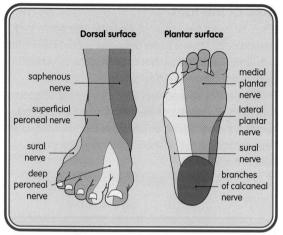

Fig. 6.39 Distribution of nerves of the foot.

Nerves of the foot

These are described in Figs 6.39 and 6.40.

Blood supply to the foot

The posterior tibial artery terminates by dividing into the medial and lateral plantar arteries (Fig. 6.41).

The medial plantar artery passes forward with the medial plantar nerve. It gives off muscular branches and terminates as a plantar digital branch to the medial side of the big toe and as branches that join the metatarsal branch of the palmar arch.

The lateral plantar artery crosses the sole of the foot and gives off muscular and cutaneous branches. At the

Fig. 6.40 Nerves of the foot.

Outline of the nerves of the foot	
Nerve (origin)	**Distribution**
saphenous (femoral nerve)	supplies skin on medial side of foot as far anteriorly as head of 1st metatarsal
superficial peroneal (common peroneal nerve)	supplies skin on dorsum of foot and all digits, except lateral side of 5th and adjoining sides of 1st and 2nd digits
deep peroneal (common peroneal nerve)	supplies extensor digitorum brevis and skin on contiguous sides of 1st and 2nd digits
medial plantar (larger terminal branch of the tibial nerve)	supplies skin of medial side of sole of foot and sides of first three digits; also supplies abductor hallucis, flexor digitorum brevis, flexor hallucis brevis, and 1st lumbrical
lateral plantar (smaller terminal branch of the tibial nerve)	supplies quadratus plantae, abductor digiti minimi and flexor digiti minimi brevis; deep branch supplies plantar and dorsal interossei, lateral three lumbricals, and adductor hallucis; supplies skin on sole lateral to a line splitting 4th digit
sural (tibial and common peroneal nerves)	lateral aspect of foot
calcaneal nerves (tibial and sural nerves)	skin of heel

level of the base of the 5th metatarsal the artery passes medially and anastomoses with the dorsalis pedis artery to form the plantar arch. From this arch plantar metatarsal arteries arise and these form the plantar digital arteries for the toes.

Arches of the foot

The foot has a longitudinal arch, which may be divided into a medial and lateral arch:

- The medial is higher than the lateral arch and consists of the calcaneus, talus, navicular, and cuneiform bones and the medial three metatarsals.
- The lower lateral arch consists of the calcaneus, the cuboid, and the lateral two metatarsals.

Functions of the feet

The feet serve to:

- Support the body weight.
- Maintain balance.
- Act as propulsive levers, e.g. in walking and running.

- Describe the skeleton of the leg and foot and the anatomy of the ankle joint.
- Outline the anatomy of the anterior and posterior compartments of the leg.
- Describe the anatomy of the dorsum of the foot and the extensor retinaculum.
- Discuss the blood and nerve supply of the sole of the foot.

transverse and oblique heads of adductor hallucis muscle

flexor hallucis brevis muscle

plantar arch

flexor digiti minimi brevis muscle

abductor hallucis muscle

lateral plantar artery and nerve

medial plantar artery and nerve

Fig. 6.41 Blood and nerve supply to the sole of the foot.

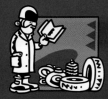

7. The Head and Neck

REGIONS AND COMPONENTS OF THE HEAD AND NECK

Skull

The skull is composed of a number of different bones joined at sutures. The bones of the skull may be divided into:

- The cranium
- The facial skeleton.

The cranium is subdivided into:

- An upper part—the vault.
- A lower part—the base of the skull.

Norma verticalis

A view of the skull from above (norma verticalis) is illustrated in Fig. 7.1.

Norma occipitalis

A view of the skull from behind (norma occipitalis) is shown in Fig. 7.2. Note the mastoid process of the temporal bone and the external occipital protuberance—a midline elevation from the occipital bone—from which the superior nuchal line extends laterally.

Norma frontalis

The skull is viewed from the front (norma frontalis) in Fig. 7.3. The frontal bones form the forehead and the superior margin of the orbits. They articulate with the nasal bones and the frontal process of the maxilla (upper jaw). The mandible (lower jaw) lies below the maxilla. Both mandible and maxilla bear teeth.

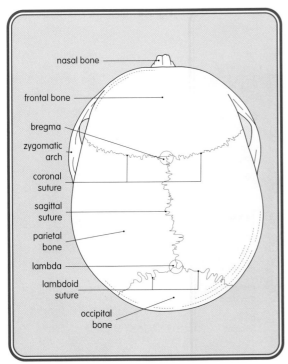

Fig. 7.1 Skull viewed from above.

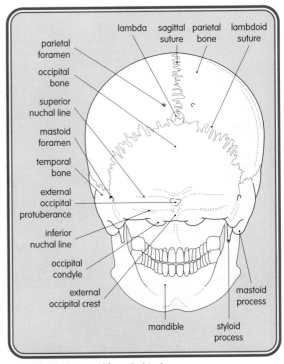

Fig. 7.2 Skull viewed from behind.

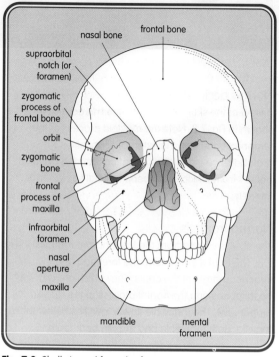

Fig. 7.3 Skull viewed from the front.

Norma lateralis

Fig. 7.4 shows the lateral view (norma lateralis) of the skull. The parietal bone articulates with the greater wing of the sphenoid bone and the temporal bone. These three bones meet at a point, the pterion, which is the thinnest part of the lateral aspect of the skull and vulnerable to damage. The middle meningeal artery lies just deep to this point and may rupture following trauma to the head.

The zygomatic arch is formed by the zygomatic process of the temporal bone and the temporal process of the zygomatic bone.

Norma basalis

In Fig. 7.5 the skull is viewed from below (norma basalis). The palate is formed by the palatine process of the maxilla and the horizontal processes of the palatine bones. The alveolar process of the maxilla surrounds the palate.

Fig. 7.4 Lateral view of the skull.

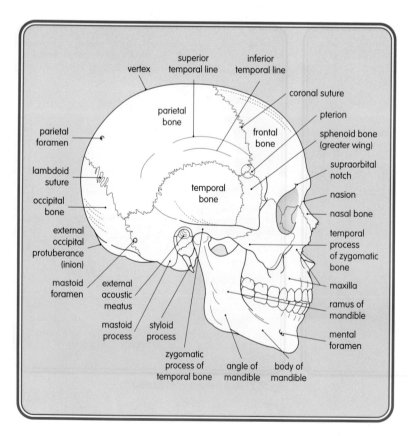

Openings in the skull

Fig. 7.6 lists the important openings in the base of the skull and their contents.

Cervical vertebrae

There are seven cervical vertebrae forming the skeleton of the neck. All except C1 (atlas), C2 (axis), and C7 are typical vertebrae (Figs 7.7 and 7.8). C7 possesses a longer spinous process, which is the most superior spinous process palpable.

Atlanto-occipital joint

This is the articulation between the the lateral masses of C1 vertebra and the occipital condyles. It is a synovial joint surrounded by a loose capsule. Flexion and extension are allowed at this joint, but no rotation.

Atlantoaxial joints

There are two lateral synovial joints between the lateral masses of the axis and atlas (Fig. 7.9). There is also a median joint between the dens (odontoid process) of the axis and the anterior arch of the atlas. These joints allow rotational movements of the head in which the skull and the atlas rotate as a unit on the axis. Alar ligaments prevent excess rotation.

The transverse ligament of the atlas holds the dens against the anterior arch of the atlas. Rupture of this ligament, e.g. during head trauma, allows the dens to impinge on the cervical spinal cord, causing paralysis of the body below the neck. If the dens compresses the medulla, the patient may die.

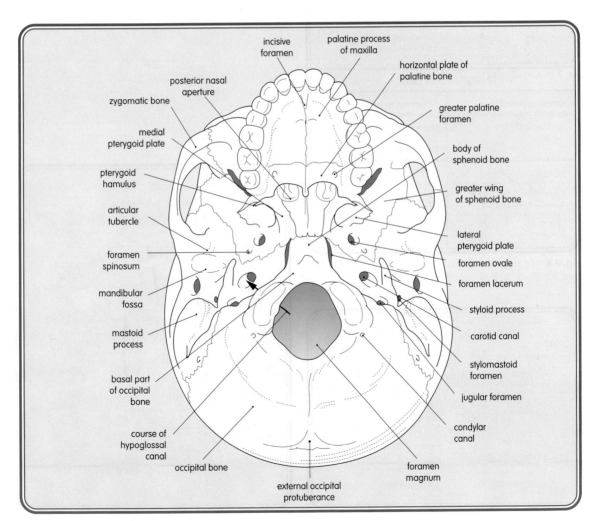

Fig. 7.5 Skull seen from below.

127

Openings in the base of the skull and structures that pass through them	
Anterior cranial fossa	
Opening in skull	**Structures transmitted**
perforations in cribriform plate	I nerve
Middle cranial fossa	
Opening in skull	**Structures transmitted**
foramen ovale	V_3, lesser petrosal nerve
foramen rotundum	V_2 nerve
foramen spinosum	middle meningeal artery
foramen lacerum	internal carotid artery
optic canal	II nerve, ophthalmic artery
superior orbital fissure	lacrimal, frontal, and nasociliary of V, IV, VI nerves; superior ophthalmic vein
Posterior cranial fossa	
Opening in skull	**Structures transmitted**
foramen magnum	medulla oblongata, spinal part of XI nerve, right and left vertebral arteries
hypoglossal canal	XII nerve
internal acoustic meatus	VII and VIII nerves
jugular foramen	IX nerve, X nerve; sigmoid sinus becomes internal jugular vein

Fig. 7.6 The important openings in the base of the skull and the structures that pass through them.

Distinctive characteristics of a typical cervical vertebra	
Part	**Characteristics**
body	small; longer from side to side than anteroposteriorly; superior surface is concave, inferior surface is convex
vertebral foramen	large and triangular
transverse processes	foramina transversaria (small or absent in C7)
articular processes	superior facets directed superoposteriorly, inferior facets directed inferoanteriorly
spinous processes	short and bifid in C3 to C5, long in C6, and longer in C7

Fig. 7.8 Distinctive characteristics of a typical cervical vertebra.

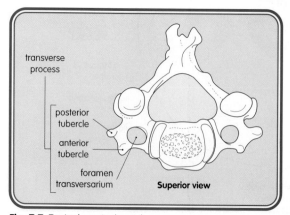

Fig. 7.7 Typical cervical vertebra.

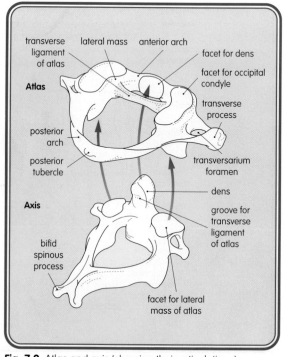

Fig. 7.9 Atlas and axis (showing their articulations).

THE FACE AND SCALP

Scalp

The scalp consists of five layers (Fig. 7.10) and has a very rich blood supply (Fig. 7.11). Injuries to this region often result in profuse bleeding.

The scalp veins follow the arterial supply:

- The supraorbital and supratrochlear veins unite to form the facial vein.
- The superficial temporal vein joins with the maxillary vein to form the retromandibular vein in the parotid salivary gland.

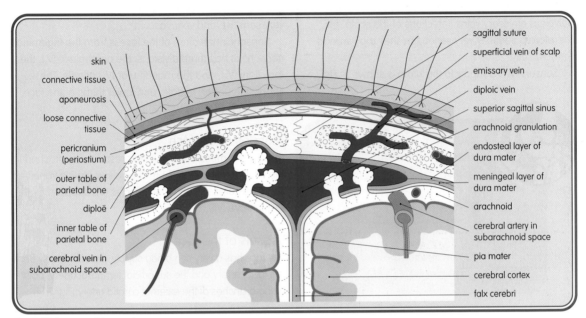

Fig. 7.10 Layers of the scalp.

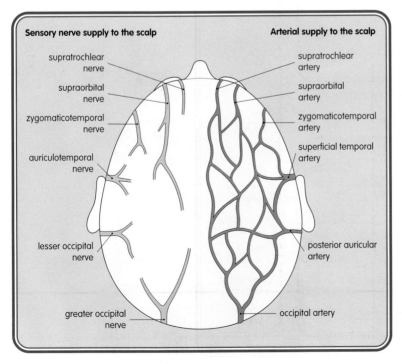

Fig. 7.11 Nerve and arterial supply to the scalp.

- The posterior auricular vein unites with the posterior division of the retromandibular vein to form the external jugular vein.
- Occipital veins drain into the suboccipital venous complex.

The scalp veins connect with the diploic veins in the skull bones and the intracranial venous sinuses by valveless emissary veins. Infections of the scalp are therefore potentially very serious as they may spread intracranially.

Sensory nerve supply to the scalp is shown in Fig.

The order of the layers of the scalp are:
S Skin
C Connective tissue
A Aponeurosis
L Loose connective tissue
P Pericranium (periostium)

7.11. The muscles of the scalp and external ear are supplied by the facial nerve.

Face

The skin of the face is connected to the facial bones by loose connective tissue. There is no deep fascia. The muscles (of facial expression) of the face lie in this connective tissue. Like the scalp, the skin of the face is very sensitive and very vascular.

Sensory innervation of the face is from the trigeminal nerve (V). It has three divisions: the ophthalmic (V_1), the maxillary (V_2), and the mandibular (V_3) nerves. These supply the upper, middle, and lower thirds of the face, respectively (Fig. 7.12).

Muscles of the face

Most of the muscles of facial expression are attached to the overlying skin (Fig. 7.13). They allow a wide variety of facial postures. All of these muscles are supplied by the facial nerve (VII).

Vessels of the face

The face has a very rich blood supply, derived mainly from the facial artery and the superficial temporal artery, both being branches of the external carotid artery (Fig. 7.14).

Fig. 7.12 Nerves of the face.

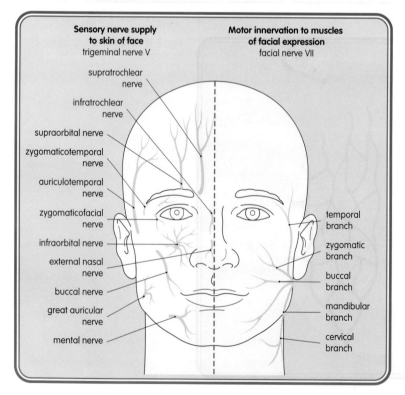

Sensory nerve supply to skin of face
trigeminal nerve V

Motor innervation to muscles of facial expression
facial nerve VII

supratrochlear nerve
infratrochlear nerve
supraorbital nerve
zygomaticotemporal nerve
auriculotemporal nerve
zygomaticofacial nerve
infraorbital nerve
external nasal nerve
buccal nerve
great auricular nerve
mental nerve

temporal branch
zygomatic branch
buccal branch
mandibular branch
cervical branch

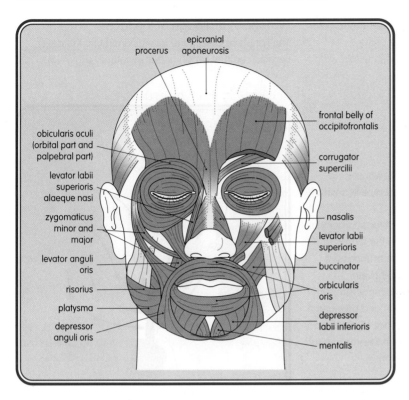

Fig. 7.13 Muscles of the face.

epicranial
aponeurosis

procerus

frontal belly of
occipitofrontalis

obicularis oculi
(orbital part and
palpebral part)

corrugator
supercilii

levator labii
superioris
alaeque nasi

nasalis

zygomaticus
minor and
major

levator labii
superioris

levator anguli
oris

buccinator

risorius

orbicularis
oris

platysma

depressor
labii inferioris

depressor
anguli oris

mentalis

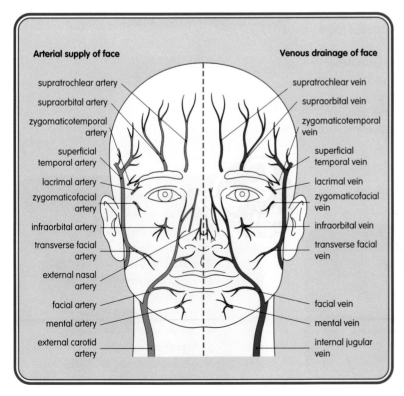

Fig. 7.14 Blood supply to the face.

Arterial supply of face

Venous drainage of face

supratrochlear artery

supratrochlear vein

supraorbital artery

supraorbital vein

zygomaticotemporal
artery

zygomaticotemporal
vein

superficial
temporal artery

superficial
temporal vein

lacrimal artery

lacrimal vein

zygomaticofacial
artery

zygomaticofacial
vein

infraorbital artery

infraorbital vein

transverse facial
artery

transverse facial
vein

external nasal
artery

facial artery

facial vein

mental artery

mental vein

external carotid
artery

internal jugular
vein

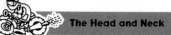

The facial artery ascends deep to the submandibular gland, winds around the inferior border of the mandible, and enters the face. It gives off the following branches as it ascends in the face:

- The inferior labial artery.
- The superior labial artery.
- The lateral nasal artery.
- The angular artery.

The supraorbital and supratrochlear arteries are terminal branches of the ophthalmic artery, a branch of the internal carotid artery.

The facial vein is formed by the union of the supraorbital and supratrochlear veins. It descends in the face and receives tributaries corresponding to the branches of the artery. It drains into the internal jugular vein.

The facial vein connects with the cavernous sinus in the skull via the superior ophthalmic vein and provides a path for spread of infection from the face to the cavernous sinus. Even minor infections in the infraorbital region may cause this grave complication.

Motor nerve supply to the face

This is from the facial nerve (VII). The nerve exits the skull through the stylomastoid foramen to lie between the ramus of the mandible and the mastoid process. It enters the parotid gland and divides into its five groups of terminal branches that supply the muscles of facial expression (see Fig. 7.12).

Before entering the parotid gland the facial nerve gives off the posterior auricular nerve and a muscular branch, which supply the occipital belly of occipitofrontalis, the stylohyoid muscle, the posterior belly of the digastric muscle, and the posterior auricular muscle.

Lymphatic drainage of the face

The lymph vessels of the face all drain into the deep cervical chain of lymph nodes eventually (Fig. 7.15).

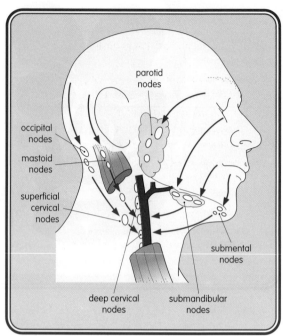

Fig. 7.15 Lymphatic drainage of the face. (Adapted from *Anatomy as a Basis for Clinical Medicine*, by E.C.B. Hall-Craggs. Courtesy of Williams & Wilkins.)

For branches of the facial nerve to the face use the following mnemonic: Ten Zulus *Bought* My Cat (temporal, zygomatic, buccal, mandibular, cervical).

- Describe the anatomy of the scalp, including its blood and nerve supply.
- Discuss the blood supply and sensory innervation of the face.
- Outline the function and nerve supply of the muscles of facial expression.

THE CRANIAL CAVITY AND MENINGES

The cranium protects the brain and its surrounding meninges. The outer surface of the cranial bones is covered by the pericranium, the inner surface by the endocranium. The two layers are continuous at the sutures of the skull and are the periosteum of the skull bones.

The cranial bones consist of outer and inner tables of compact bones separated by cancellous bone containing red marrow, the diploë (see Fig. 7.10).

The base of the skull forms the floor on which the brain lies. The internal surface of the base may be divided into the anterior, middle, and posterior cranial fossae (Fig. 7.16).

Cranial fossae
Anterior cranial fossa
The olfactory nerves perforate the cribriform plate of the ethmoid bone. The anterior ethmoidal nerve passes through a small slit in this bone. The crista galli projects upwards from the cribriform plate.

The anterior cranial fossa contains the frontal lobes of the brain and the olfactory bulbs.

Middle cranial fossa
A shallow depression near the apex of the petrous temporal bone houses the trigeminal ganglion.

The middle cranial fossa contains the temporal lobes of the cerebral hemispheres, the floor of the forebrain, the optic chiasma, the termination of the internal carotid arteries, and the pituitary gland.

The pituitary gland lies in the pituitary fossa or sella turcica, below the optic chiasma. A tumour of the pituitary gland may compress the chiasma. As this carries fibres from the temporal fields, the patient will complain of 'tunnel vision' or a bitemporal hemianopia.

Posterior cranial fossa
This is roofed by the tentorium cerebelli layer of the dura mater. It contains the pons, the medulla, the cerebellum, and the midbrain.

The foramina in the cranial fossae are outlined in Fig. 7.6.

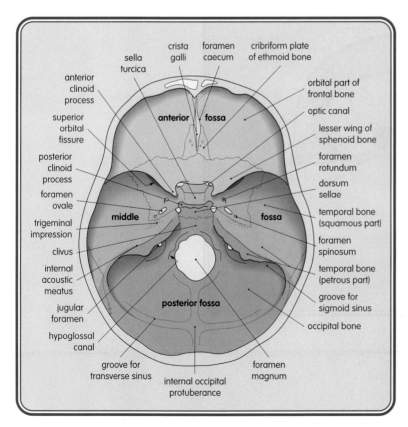

Fig. 7.16 Internal surface of the base of the skull, showing the cranial fossae.

Meninges

There are three meningeal layers surrounding the brain and spinal cord (see Fig. 7.10):

- The dura mater.
- The arachnoid mater.
- The pia mater.

Dura mater

This may be divided into two layers:

- The endosteal layer is the endosteum (periosteum) lining the inner surface of the cranial bones.
- The meningeal layer (the dura mater proper) is made up of dense strong fibrous tissue. It is continuous with the dura mater of the spinal cord through the foramen magnum. The dura sends sheets around the cranial nerves which fuse with the epineurium of the nerves outside the skull.

The meningeal layer of dura mater gives rise to four septa that assist in restricting rotatory displacement of the brain:

- The falx cerebri.
- The tentorium cerebelli.
- The falx cerebelli.
- The diaphragma sellae.

Falx cerebri

This is a sickle-shaped fold of dura lying in the midline between the two cerebral hemispheres (Fig. 7.17). It is attached anteriorly to the internal frontal crest and the crista galli. Posteriorly it blends with the tentorium cerebelli.

The superior sagittal sinus runs in its superior margin, which is its attachment to the vault of the skull. The inferior sagittal sinus runs in its inferior margin. The straight sinus runs along its attachment to the tentorium cerebelli.

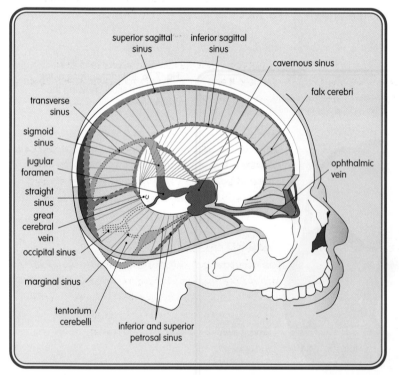

Fig. 7.17 Positions of the cranial venous sinuses, falx cerebri, and tentorium cerebelli.

Tentorium cerebelli
This is a crescent-shaped fold of dura mater that roofs the posterior cranial fossa (see Fig. 7.17). It covers the cerebellum and supports the occipital lobes of the cerebral hemispheres. The midbrain passes through the tentorial notch anteriorly.

The tentorium is attached to the anterior clinoid process anteriorly. Posteriorly the falx cerebri and falx cerebelli are attached to its upper and lower surfaces.

The superior petrosal and transverse venous sinuses run along its attachment to the petrous and occipital bones, respectively.

Falx cerebelli
This is a small fold of dura mater attached to the internal occipital crest. It projects forward between the two cerebellar hemispheres. Its posterior margin contains the occipital sinus.

Diaphragma sellae
This is a small circular fold of dura forming the roof of the pituitary fossa.

Arachnoid mater
This surrounds the brain. It is separated from the dura mater by the subdural (potential) space and from the pia mater by the subarachnoid space, which contains cerebrospinal fluid.

Where the arachnoid bridges major irregularities of the brain surface, the space expands to form subarachnoid cisterns.

Pia mater
This closely invests the brain surface. It continues as a sheath around the small vessels entering the brain. In some areas the pia invaginates into the ventricles to take part in the formation of the choroid plexus, which secretes cerebrospinal fluid.

Nerve supply of the meninges
Dura mater in the anterior and middle cranial fossae is supplied by the trigeminal nerve; in the posterior fossa it is supplied by the upper three cervical nerves.

Cranial venous sinuses
These lie between the endosteal and meningeal layers of dura mater, are lined by endothelium, and are valveless (see Fig. 7.17). Tributaries from the various parts of the brain and from the diploë, the orbit, and the inner ear drain into these sinuses.

Superior sagittal sinus
This runs in the upper border of the falx cerebri. It commences at the foramen caecum and passes backwards, grooving the vault of the skull. At the internal occipital protuberance it dilates to form the confluence of the sinuses and continues as a transverse sinus (usually the right). It receives the occipital sinus and numerous cerebral veins and shows several accumulations of arachnoid granulations (see Fig. 7.10).

Inferior sagittal sinus
This lies in the free margin of the falx cerebri. At the free margin of the tentorium cerebelli it joins the great cerebral vein to form the straight sinus.

Straight sinus
This lies between the falx cerebri and tentorium cerebelli. It ends by turning to form a transverse sinus (usually to the left).

Transverse sinuses
These commence at the internal occipital protuberance and run in the attachment of the tentorium cerebelli. They end by turning inferiorly as the sigmoid sinuses. They receive the superior petrosal sinuses and the cerebral, cerebellar, and diploic veins.

Sigmoid sinuses
Each sinus turns downward and medially to groove the mastoid process, lying behind the mastoid antrum. It then turns downward through the posterior part of the jugular foramen to become continuous with the superior bulb of the internal jugular vein.

Occipital sinus

This lies in the attached margin of the falx cerebelli. It drains into the confluence of sinuses.

Cavernous sinuses

These lie on either side of the body of the sphenoid and extend from the superior orbital fissure anteriorly to the apex of the petrous temporal bone posteriorly.

They receive:

- The superior and inferior ophthalmic veins.
- The cerebral veins.
- The sphenoparietal sinus.
- The central vein of the retina.

They drain posteriorly into the superior and inferior petrosal sinuses and inferiorly into the pterygoid venous plexus. The two sinuses communicate via anterior and posterior intercavernous sinuses.

Relations of the cavenous sinuses

The internal carotid artery and its sympathetic nerve plexus and the abducens nerve run through the sinus (Fig. 7.18). The oculomotor and trochlear nerves and the ophthalmic and maxillary divisions of the trigeminal nerves lie in the lateral wall of the sinus, between the endothelium and the dura.

Superior and inferior petrosal sinuses

These lie at the superior and inferior borders of the petrous temporal bone, respectively.

Each superior sinus drains the cavernous sinus into the transverse sinus. Each inferior sinus drains the cavernous sinus into the internal jugular vein.

Arteries of the cranial cavity

The brain is supplied by the two internal carotid arteries and the two vertebral arteries.

Internal carotid artery

This is a terminal branch of the common carotid artery (Fig. 7.19). It enters the skull through the carotid canal and enters the middle cranial fossa through the foramen lacerum in the floor of the cavernous sinus. The artery runs forward in the cavernous sinus. At the anterior end of the sinus it turns superiorly and pierces the roof. It then enters the subarachnoid space and turns backwards to the region of the anterior perforated substance of the brain at the medial end of the lateral cerebral sulcus. Here it divides into the anterior and middle cerebral arteries.

Branches of the internal carotid include:

- The ophthalmic artery.
- The posterior communicating artery.

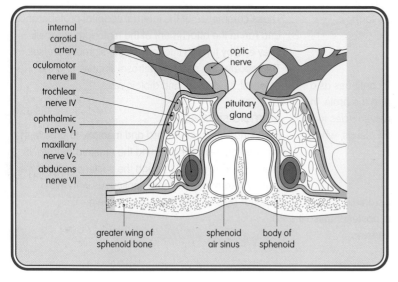

Fig. 7.18 Cavernous sinus and its relations.

internal carotid artery

oculomotor nerve III

trochlear nerve IV

ophthalmic nerve V$_1$

maxillary nerve V$_2$

abducens nerve VI

optic nerve

pituitary gland

greater wing of sphenoid bone

sphenoid air sinus

body of sphenoid

- The choroidal artery.
- The anterior cerebral artery.
- The middle cerebral artery.

Vertebral artery

This arises from the first part of the subclavian artery (see Fig. 7.19). It ascends in the foramina of the upper six cervical vertebrae transverse processes and enters the skull through the foramen magnum. It passes upwards on the medulla oblongata and joins the vessel from the opposite side to form the basilar artery.

Cranial branches of the vertebral artery include:
- The meningeal arteries.
- The anterior and posterior spinal arteries.
- The posterior inferior cerebellar artery.
- The medullary arteries.

Basilar artery

This ascends on the anterior border of the pons (see Fig. 7.19). At the upper border of the pons it divides into the posterior cerebral arteries. It also gives off branches to the pons, cerebellum, and internal ear.

Circus arteriosus

This is an anastomosis between branches of the internal carotid arteries and the vertebral arteries (see Fig. 7.19). It lies in the interpeduncular fossa beneath the forebrain. It allows blood entering either the carotid or vertebral artery to flow to any part of both cerebral hemispheres.

Strokes or cerebrovascular accidents are common in Western countries. They commonly arise because of blockage of one of the major arteries, usually the middle cerebral artery. The anastomosis between the cerebral vessels is not sufficient to supply the affected tissue, resulting in death of that part of the brain.

Cranial nerves

These are summarized in Fig. 7.20.

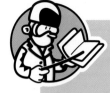

- Outline the structure and contents of the anterior, middle, and posterior cranial fossae.
- Describe the anatomy of the meninges.
- Discuss the anatomy of the cranial venous sinuses.
- Describe the anatomy of the cranial nerves.
- Summarize the circus arteriosus and the main vessels of the skull.

anterior cerebral artery
optic chiasma
internal carotid artery
middle cerebral artery
posterior communicating artery
oculomotor nerve
posterior cerebral artery
superior cerebellar artery
pontine arteries
labyrinthine artery
posterior inferior cerebellar artery
anterior spinal artery

anterior communicating artery
central branches
base of the brain

basilar artery
anterior inferior cerebellar artery
vertebral artery

Fig. 7.19 Internal carotid and vertebral arteries.

Summary of cranial nerves	
Nerve	**Distribution and functions**
olfactory (I)	smell from nasal mucosa of roof of each nasal cavity
optic (II)	vision from retina
oculomotor (III)	motor to all extrinsic eye muscles except superior oblique and lateral rectus; parasympathetic innervation to sphincter pupillae and ciliary muscle (constricts pupil and accommodates lens of eye)
trochlear (IV)	motor to superior oblique
trigeminal (V) —ophthalmic division (V_1)	sensation from upper third of face, including cornea, scalp, eyelids, and paranasal sinuses
trigeminal (V) —maxillary division (V_2)	sensation from the middle third of face, including upper lip, maxillary teeth, mucosa of nose, maxillary sinuses, and palate
trigeminal (V) —mandibular division (V_3)	motor to muscles of mastication, mylohyoid, anterior belly of digastric, tensor veli palatini and tensor tympani; sensation from lower third of face, including temporomandibular joint, and mucosa of mouth and anterior two-thirds of tongue
abducent (VI)	motor to lateral rectus
facial (VII)	motor to muscles of facial expression and scalp, stapedius, stylohyoid, and posterior belly of digastric; taste from anterior two-thirds of tongue, floor of mouth, and palate; sensation from skin of external acoustic meatus; parasympathetic innervation to submandibular and sublingual salivary glands, lacrimal gland, and glands of nose and palate
vestibulocochlear (VIII)	vestibular sensation from semicircular ducts, utricle, and saccule; hearing from spiral organ
glossopharyngeal (IX)	motor to stylopharyngeus, parasympathetic innervation to parotid gland; visceral sensation from parotid gland, carotid body and sinus, pharynx, and middle ear; taste and general sensation from posterior third of tongue; cutaneous sensation from external ear
vagus (X)	motor to constrictor muscles of pharynx, intrinsic muscles of larynx, and muscles of palate (except tensor veli palatini) and superior two-thirds of oesophagus; parasympathetic innervation to smooth muscle of trachea, bronchi, digestive tract, and cardiac muscle of heart; visceral sensation from pharynx, larynx, trachea, bronchi, heart, oesophagus, stomach, and intestine; taste from epiglottis and palate; sensation from auricle, external acoustic meatus, and dura mater of posterior cranial fossa
accessory (XI) cranial root spinal root	motor to striated muscles of soft palate, pharynx, and larynx via fibres that join X in jugular foramen motor to sternocleidomastoid and trapezius
hypoglossal (XII)	motor to muscles of tongue (except palatoglossus)

Fig. 7.20 Cranial nerves.

THE ORBIT

The eyeball and its associated muscles, nerves, and vessels are protected by the bony orbital cavity. The mobile eyelids protect the eyes anteriorly.

Eyelids

The eyelids are two mobile folds of skin lying in front of the eye and separated by the palpebral fissure (Fig. 7.21). The superficial surface of the lids is covered by the skin; the deep surface is covered by mucosa, the conjunctiva.

Sebaceous, ciliary, and tarsal glands pour their secretions onto the eyelid.

The medial angle of the eye is the lacus lacrimalis. It contains an elevation, the caruncle lacrimalis. Tears produced by the lacrimal gland are continually spread over the conjunctiva and cornea by blinking, preventing damage to the eye. The tears are then forced towards the lacus lacrimalis and pass through the puncta lacrimalia to enter the canaliculi lacrimales, which drain into the lacrimal sac. This sac is the upper blind end of the nasolacrimal duct, which drains the tears into the inferior meatus of the nose.

The nerve supply to the lacrimal gland is parasympathetic secretomotor, which originates in the lacrimal ganglion and reaches the gland via the pterygopalatine ganglion.

The fibrous framework of the eyelids is formed by the orbital septum (Fig. 7.22). This is thickened at the lid margins to form the tarsal plates, which medially and laterally form the medial palpebral ligament and the lateral palpebral raphe, respectively. The levator palpebrae superioris muscle is attached to the superior tarsal plate.

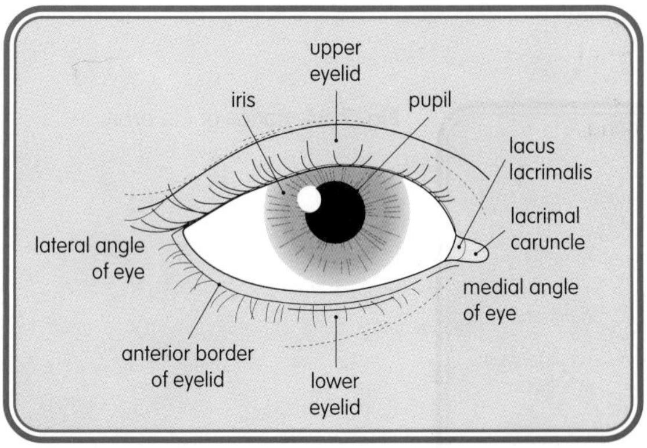

Fig. 7.21 Eyelids, palpebral fissure, and eyeball.

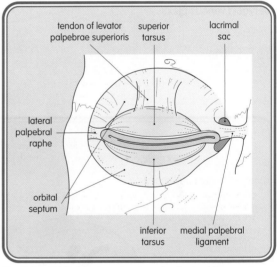

Fig. 7.22 Orbital septum, tarsi, and palpebral ligaments.

The conjunctiva is the mucous membrane lining the eyelid. It is reflected at the superior and inferior fornices onto the anterior surface of the eyeball, forming the conjunctival sac when the eyes are closed (Fig. 7.23).

Orbital cavity

Fig. 7.24 illustrates the bony components of the orbital cavity. Fig. 7.25 shows the orbital openings and their contents.

Muscles of the orbit

These are outlined in Fig. 7.26 and illustrated in Fig. 7.27.

Vessels of the orbit

Fig. 7.28 shows the arterial supply to the orbit.

The superior ophthalmic vein communicates anteriorly with the facial vein and posteriorly drains to the cavernous sinus. The inferior ophthalmic vein communicates via the inferior orbital fissure with the pterygoid venous plexus.

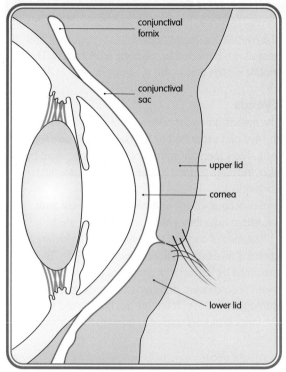

Fig. 7.23 Conjunctival sac, upper and lower lids, and cornea.

Fig. 7.24 Bones of the orbit.

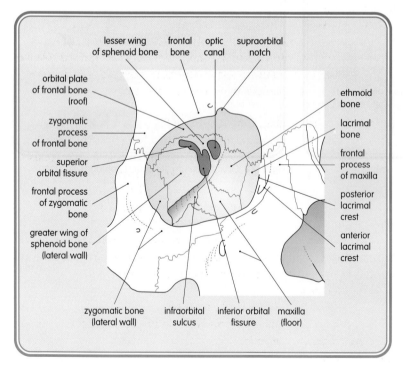

Orbital openings and their contents		
Openings	**Bones**	**Contents**
supraorbital notch (foramen)	orbital plate of the frontal bone	supraorbital nerve and vessels
infraorbital groove and canal	orbital plate of the maxilla	infraorbital nerve and vessels
inferior orbital fissure	maxilla and greater wing of the sphenoid bone	communicates with the pterygopalatine fossa and transmits the maxillary nerve and its zygomatic branch, the inferior ophthalmic vein, and sympathetic nerves
superior orbital fissure	greater and lesser wing of the sphenoid bone	lacrimal, frontal, trochlear, oculomotor, and nasociliary nerves, and superior ophthalmic vein
optic canal	lesser wing of the sphenoid bone	optic nerve and ophthalmic artery
zygomaticotemporal and zygomaticofacial foramina	zygomatic bone	zygomaticotemporal and zygomaticofacial nerves
anterior and posterior ethmoidal foramina	ethmoid bone	anterior and posterior ethmoidal nerves

Fig. 7.25 Orbital openings and their contents.

Nerves of the orbit

Optic nerve (II)

This is surrounded by the three meningeal layers as it enters the orbit. It runs forward and laterally within the cone of rectus muscles and pierces the sclera. The meningeal layer fuses with the sclera here. The nerve carries afferent fibres from the retina.

Lacrimal nerve

This is a branch of the ophthalmic division of the trigeminal nerve (V$_1$). It passes along the upper part of the lateral rectus muscle to supply the skin of the upper lid laterally. It is joined by a branch of the zygomaticotemporal nerve carrying parasympathetic fibres to the lacrimal gland.

Frontal nerve

This is also a branch of V$_3$. It passes forward on the superior surface of levator palpebrae superioris. Just before it reaches the orbital margin it divides into the supraorbital and supratrochlear nerves, which supply the skin of the forehead and scalp and the frontal sinus.

Nasociliary nerve

Another branch of V$_3$, this enters the orbit and crosses above the optic nerve with the ophthalmic artery to reach the medial wall of the orbit. It runs forward on the upper margin of medial rectus and ends by dividing into the anterior ethmoidal and infratrochlear nerves (Fig. 7.29).

Trochlear nerve (IV)   SO4

This leaves the lateral wall of the cavernous sinus to enter the orbit. It runs forward and medially across the origin of levator palpebrae superioris to the superior oblique muscle which it supplies.

Oculomotor nerve (III)   (LR$_6$SO$_4$)$_3$

This is divided into superior and inferior divisions:

- The superior division supplies the superior rectus and levator palpebrae superioris.
- The inferior division supplies the inferior rectus, medial rectus, and inferior oblique.

The nerve to inferior oblique sends a branch to the ciliary ganglion. This carries parasympathetic fibres to the sphincter pupillae and ciliary muscle.

Abducent nerve (VI)

This enters the orbit and supplies the lateral rectus muscle.   LR$_6$

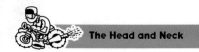

4 Recti, 2 oblique   **Muscles of the eyeballs and eyelids**

Extrinsic muscles of eyeball (striated skeletal muscle)

Name of muscle (nerve supply)	Origin	Insertion	Action
superior rectus (III nerve)	common tendinous ring on posterior wall of orbital cavity	superior surface of eyeball just posterior to corneoscleral junction	raises eyeball upward and medially
inferior rectus (III nerve)	common tendinous ring on posterior wall of orbital cavity	inferior surface of eyeball just posterior to corneoscleral junction	depresses eyeball downward and medially
medial rectus (III nerve)	common tendinous ring on posterior wall of orbital cavity	medial surface of eyeball just posterior to corneoscleral junction	rotates eyeball so that cornea looks medially
lateral rectus (VI nerve)	common tendinous ring on posterior wall of orbital cavity	lateral surface of eyeball just posterior to corneoscleral junction	rotates eyeball so that cornea looks laterally
superior oblique (IV nerve)	posterior wall of orbital cavity	passes through trochlea and is attached to superior surface of eyeball beneath superior rectus	rotates eyeball so that cornea looks downward and laterally
inferior oblique (III nerve)	floor of orbital cavity	lateral surface of eyeball deep to lateral rectus	rotates eyeball so that cornea looks upward and laterally

Intrinsic muscles of eyeball (smooth muscle)

Name of muscle (nerve supply)	Origin	Insertion	Action
sphincter pupillae of iris (parasympathetic via III nerve)	–	–	constricts pupil
dilator pupillae of iris (sympathetic)	–	–	dilates pupil
ciliary muscle (parasympathetic via III nerve)	–	–	controls shape of lens; in accommodation, makes lens more globular

Muscles of eyelids

Name of muscle (nerve supply)	Origin	Insertion	Action
orbicularis oculi	(see Fig. 7.13)		
levator palpebrae superioris (striated muscle: III nerve; smooth muscle: sympathetic)	back of orbital cavity	superior tarsal plate	raises upper lid

Fig. 7.26 Muscles of the eyeballs and eyelids.

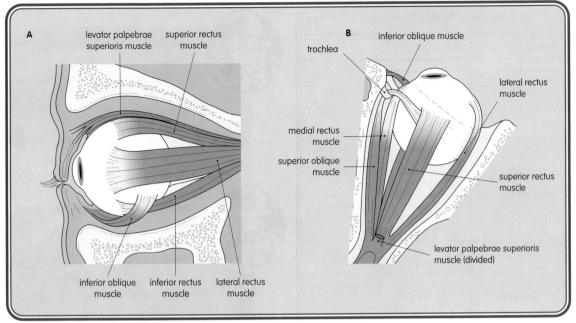

Fig. 7.27 Muscles of the orbit seen from above (A) and below (B).

Fig. 7.28 Arterial supply to the orbit.

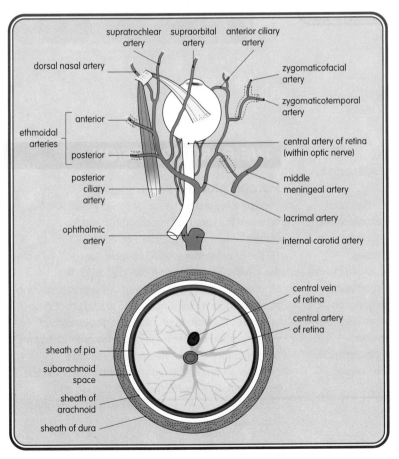

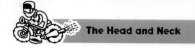

Branches of the nasociliary nerve	
Branch	**Action**
communicating branch	communicates with the ciliary ganglion—sensory fibres from the eyeball pass to the ciliary ganglion via the short ciliary nerves and then to the nasociliary nerve via the communicating branch
long ciliary nerve	2–3 branches containing sympathetic fibres for the dilator pupillae—runs with the short ciliary nerves and pierces the sclera to reach the iris
posterior ethmoidal nerve	exits through the posterior ethmoidal foramen to supply the ethmoidal and sphenoidal air sinuses
infratrochlear nerve	passes below the trochlea to supply the skin over the upper eyelid
anterior ethmoidal nerve	exits via the anterior ethmoidal foramen and enters the anterior cranial fossa on the cribriform plate of the ethmoid; then enters the nasal cavity via an opening opposite the crista galli to supply the mucosa of the nose; then supplies the skin of the nose as the external nasal nerve

Fig. 7.29 Branches of the nasociliary nerve.

Motor innervation of the orbit is from the oculomotor nerve except for SO 4 and LR 6 (superior oblique—IV nerve; lateral rectus—VI nerve).

- Describe the anatomy of the eyelids and lacrimal apparatus.
- Discuss the muscles and the blood and nerve supply of the orbit, including the ciliary ganglion.
- Outline the structures passing through the foramina of the orbit.

Ciliary ganglion

This is a parasympathetic ganglion situated posteriorly in the orbit, lateral to the optic nerve.

Preganglionic fibres from the Edinger–Westphal nucleus pass to the ganglion via the oculomotor nerve.

Postganglionic parasympathetic fibres pass to the back of the eyeball via the short ciliary nerves.

Sympathetic fibres (from the internal carotid plexus) pass through the ganglion to enter the short ciliary nerves. General sensory fibres leave the ganglion via the nasociliary nerve. The long ciliary nerve also carries sympathetic and sensory fibres to the eyeball.

The parasympathetic nerves supply the constrictor pupillae; the sympathetic fibres supply the dilator pupillae.

THE PAROTID REGION

Parotid gland

This is the largest of the major salivary glands. It lies between the ramus of the mandible and the sternocleidomastoid muscle (Fig. 7.30).

The gland is surrounded by a capsule derived from the investing layer of deep cervical fascia. The stylomandibular ligament is part of the fascia, running from the mandibular angle to the styloid process. It separates the parotid and submandibular glands.

The parotid duct emerges from the anterior border of the gland. It crosses the masseter muscle superficially and at the anterior border of this muscle turns medially to pierce the buccal fat pad and buccinator to open into the oral cavity opposite the upper second molar tooth.

Structures within the parotid gland

These are shown in Fig. 7.31.

Facial nerve (VII)

This emerges from the stylomastoid foramen to enter the gland after giving off the posterior auricular nerve and muscular branches. It divides into its five terminal branches in the parotid gland.

Retromandibular vein

This is formed in the gland by the union of the superficial temporal and maxillary veins. It divides into anterior and posterior divisions, which leave the lower border of the gland. The anterior division joins the facial vein; the posterior division joins with the posterior auricular vein to form the external jugular vein.

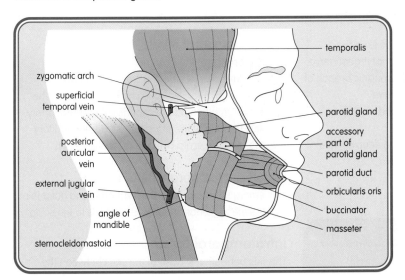

Fig. 7.30 Parotid gland and its relations. (Adapted from *Clinical Anatomy, An Illustrated Review with Questions and Explanations 2e*, by R.S. Snell. Courtesy of Churchill Livingstone.)

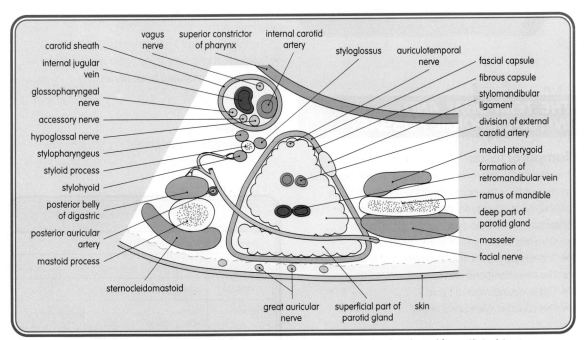

Fig. 7.31 Horizontal section of the neck, showing structures within the parotid gland. (Adapted from *Clinical Anatomy, An Illustrated Review with Questions and Explanations 2e*, by R.S. Snell. Courtesy of Churchill Livingstone.)

External carotid artery

This enters the parotid gland by passing up from the carotid triangle. At the neck of the mandible it divides into its two terminal branches—the maxillary and superficial temporal arteries.

Blood supply, lymphatic drainage, and innervation of the parotid gland

Blood supply is from the external carotid artery and its terminal branches.

Parasympathetic secretomotor fibres from the inferior salivary nucleus of the glossopharyngeal nerve (IX) pass to the otic ganglion via the tympanic branch of the IX nerve and the lesser petrosal nerve. Postganglionic fibres pass to the parotid via the auriculotemporal nerve.

Parotid nodes drain the gland to the deep cervical nodes.

○ **Describe the anatomy of the parotid gland and the structures passing through it.**

THE TEMPORAL AND INFRATEMPORAL FOSSAE

Temporal fossa

This lies on the lateral aspect of the skull. It is bounded by the superior temporal line of the temporal bone superiorly, by the frontal process of the zygomatic bone anteriorly, and by the zygomatic arch inferiorly.

Contents of the temporal fossa comprise:
- The temporalis muscle and temporal fascia.
- The deep temporal nerves and vessels.
- The auriculotemporal nerve.
- The superficial temporal artery.

Temporal fascia

This covers the temporalis muscle above the zygomatic arch. It is attached inferiorly to the zygomatic arch and superiorly to the superior temporal line.

Deep temporal nerves

Two or three nerves on each side arise from the mandibular nerve and emerge from the upper border of lateral pterygoid to enter and supply the temporalis muscle.

Deep temporal arteries

These are branches of the maxillary artery. They accompany the deep temporal nerves.

Auriculotemporal nerve

This is a branch of the posterior division of the mandibular nerve. It emerges from behind the temporomandibular joint and crosses the root of the zygomatic arch behind the superficial temporal artery. It supplies the skin of the auricle, the external auditory meatus, and the scalp over the temporal region

Superficial temporal artery

This emerges from behind the temporomandibular joint, crosses the zygomatic arch, and ascends to the scalp.

Infratemporal fossa

This lies beneath the base of the skull between the pharynx and the ramus of the mandible (Fig. 7.32). It communicates with the temporal region deep to the zygomatic arch.

The infratemporal fossa contains (Fig. 7.33):
- The medial and lateral pterygoid muscles.
- Branches of the mandibular nerve.
- The otic ganglion.
- The chorda tympani.
- The maxillary artery.
- The pterygoid venous plexus.

Boundaries of the infratemporal fossa	
Boundary	**Components**
anterior	posterior surface of the maxilla
posterior	styloid process
superior	infratemporal surface of the greater wing of the sphenoid bone
medial	lateral pterygoid plate
lateral	ramus of the mandible

Fig. 7.32 Boundaries of the infratemporal fossa.

Mandible

Important features of the mandible are shown in Fig. 7.34. The two halves of the mandible unite at the midline symphysis menti.

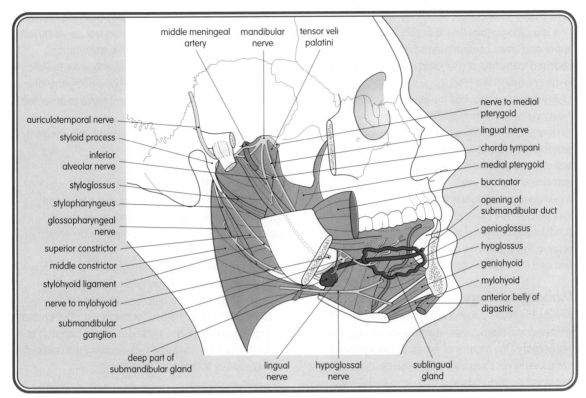

Fig. 7.33 Infratemporal fossa and its relations.

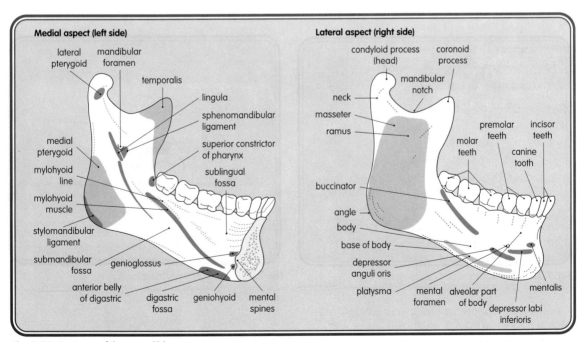

Fig. 7.34 Features of the mandible.

Temporomandibular joint

This is the articulation between the condylar head of the mandible and the mandibular fossa of the temporal bone (Figs 7.35 and 7.36).

It is a synovial joint. The joint space is divided into upper and lower compartments by an articular disc attached to the lateral pterygoid muscle anteriorly and to the capsule of the joint.

The capsule surrounds the joint and is attached to the margins of the mandibular fossa and the neck of the mandible. It is strengthened by the lateral temporomandibular ligament. The sphenomandibular and stylomandibular ligaments are also functionally associated with the joint.

Hinge-like movements (elevation and depression) take place in the lower joint space (between the condyle and the articular disc). Gliding movements occur in the upper joint space (between the articular disc and the mandibular fossa).

Mandibular nerve

V_3 exits the skull through the foramen ovale to enter the infratemporal fossa, where it immediately joins the motor root of the trigeminal nerve. Below the foramen ovale the nerve is separated from the pharynx by the tensor veli palatini muscle and is deep to the superior head of the lateral pterygoid muscle. It divides into anterior and posterior divisions (Fig. 7.37).

Otic ganglion

This is a parasympathetic ganglion lying below the foramen ovale.

Preganglionic secretomotor fibres from the inferior salivary nucleus of the glossopharyngeal nerve (IX) join the tympanic branch of the IX nerve, the tympanic plexus, and the lesser petrosal nerve to enter the otic ganglion. Here the fibres synapse and postganglionic fibres pass via the auriculotemporal nerve to enter the parotid gland.

Sympathetic fibres also pass through the ganglion, but without synapsing.

Chorda tympani

This is a branch of the facial nerve in the temporal bone. It enters the infratemporal fossa via the petrotympanic fissure and joins the lingual nerve.

It transmits:

- Preganglionic parasympathetic secretomotor fibres to the submandibular ganglion.
- Taste fibres from the anterior two-thirds of the tongue and from the floor of the mouth. Cell bodies of the taste fibres are in the geniculate ganglion of the facial nerve and end by synapsing with cells of the nucleus solitarius in the pons.

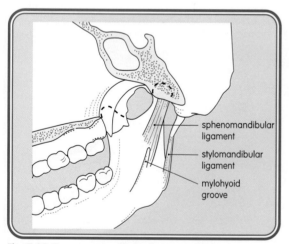

Fig. 7.35 Temporomandibular ligaments.

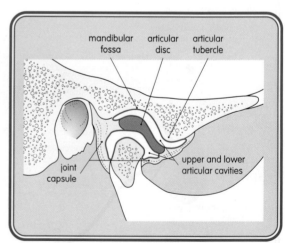

Fig. 7.36 Temporomandibular joint.

Fig. 7.37 Branches of the
mandibular nerve and the areas
they supply.

Branches of the mandibular nerve	
Branch	**Area supplied**
Main trunk	
meningeal branch	re-enters cranial cavity via foramen spinosum
nerve to medial pterygoid	medial pterygoid and a branch that passes through otic ganglion to supply tensor tympani and tensor veli palatini
Anterior division (motor except the buccal nerve)	
deep temporal nerves	temporalis muscle (see temporal region)
masseteric nerve	passes through mandibular notch to supply masseter muscle
nerve to lateral pterygoid	enters deep surface of lateral pterygoid and supplies it
buccal nerve	passes anteriorly between heads of lateral pterygoid to appear at anterior border of masseter; is sensory to skin of cheek and underlying buccal mucosa and gingiva
Posterior division (mainly sensory)	
lingual nerve	appears at lower border of lateral pterygoid and runs over superior surface of medial pterygoid to lie just beneath mucosa lining inner aspect of mandible adjacent to 3rd molar tooth (its subsequent course is described later); deep to lateral pterygoid, the nerve receives the chorda tympani
inferior alveolar nerve	runs parallel with lingual nerve over medial pterygoid; enters mandibular foramen and supplies teeth of lower jaw; at mental foramen, a branch of the nerve, the mental nerve, exits mandible to supply lower lip and chin region; mylohyoid nerve arises from inferior alveolar nerve just above mandibular foramen to supply mylohyoid and anterior belly of digastric
auriculotemporal nerve	see temporal region

Maxillary artery

This is the large terminal branch of the external carotid artery in the parotid gland. It runs forward medial to the neck of the mandible to the lower border of lateral pterygoid, entering the infratemporal fossa. It then passes between the heads of lateral pterygoid and enters the pterygopalatine fossa through the pterygomaxillary fissure. Fig. 7.38 shows the branches of the maxillary artery.

Pterygoid venous plexus

This lies around the muscles of mastication in the infratemporal fossa. It drains veins from the orbit, oral cavity, and nasal cavity. It communicates with the cavernous sinus and with the facial vein.

Branches of the maxillary artery		
Branch	**Site of origin**	**Area supplied**
deep auricular artery	behind neck of mandible	external auditory meatus and outer surface of eardrum
anterior tympanic artery	behind neck of mandible	inner surface of eardrum
middle meningeal artery	infratemporal fossa	enters cranial cavity via foramen spinosum to supply meninges
inferior alveolar artery	infratemporal fossa	follows inferior alveolar nerve into mandibular canal and supplies lower jaw and teeth, and surrounding mucosa
deep temporal arteries masseteric artery pterygoid branches	infratemporal fossa	muscles of mastication
posterior superior alveolar artery	pterygopalatine fossa	enters posterior aspect of maxilla to supply molar and premolar teeth of maxilla
infraorbital artery	pterygopalatine fossa	accompanies infraorbital nerve through infraorbital foramen onto face; reaches foramen by passing forward in infraorbital canal in orbital floor
anterior superior alveolar artery	infraorbital canal	incisor and canine teeth
palatine sphenopalatine pharyngeal branches	pterygopalatine fossa	described with the nasal cavity

Fig. 7.38 Branches of the maxillary artery.

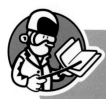

- List the muscles, blood vessels, and nerves of the temporal fossa.
- Discuss the boundaries and contents of the infratemporal fossa.
- Describe the anatomy of the mandible and the temporomandibular joint.

THE EAR AND VESTIBULAR APPARATUS

The ear is the organ of hearing and balance. It may be divided into the external ear, the middle ear, and the internal ear.

External ear
Auricle
This is a double layer of skin reinforced by cartilage. It collects sound and conducts it to the tympanic membrane.

External auditory (acoustic) meatus
This extends from the auricle to the tympanic membrane (Fig. 7.39). The lateral third is cartilaginous and the medial two-thirds are bony. It is lined by a layer of thin skin. Ceruminous and sebaceous glands produce cerumen (wax).

Tympanic membrane
This is a thin membrane lying betwen the external and middle ears (see Fig. 7.39). It is covered by skin externally and by mucous membrane internally. The membrane shows a concavity towards the meatus, with a central depression—the umbo.

The membrane moves in response to air vibration. Movements are transmitted by the ossicles through the middle ear to the internal ear.

The auriculotemporal nerve supplies the external surface of the tympanic membrane. The glossopharyngeal nerve supplies the internal surface.

Middle ear
This lies in the petrous temporal bone. It consists of the tympanic cavity and the epitympanic recess, which lies superior to the tympanic cavity.

It is connected to the nasopharynx via the auditory tube and to the mastoid air cells via the mastoid

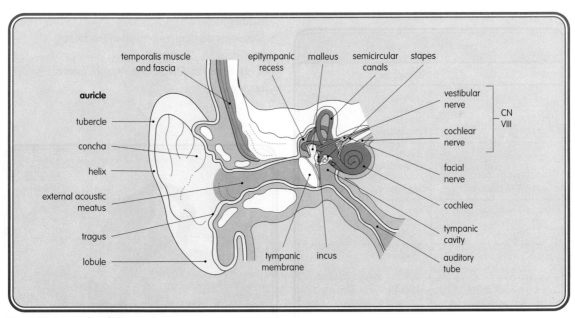

Fig. 7.39 External auditory meatus.

antrum. The mucosa lining the tympanic cavity is continuous with that of the auditory tube, mastoid cells, and the mastoid antrum.

The middle ear contains:
- The ossicles (malleus, incus, and stapes).
- Stapedius and tensor tympani muscles.
- The chorda tympani.
- The tympanic plexus of nerves.

Fig. 7.40 describes the walls of the middle ear.

Mastoid antrum

The aditus to the antrum connects the mastoid antrum to the epitympanic recess of the tympanic cavity. The tegmen tympani separates the antrum from the middle cranial fossa. The floor of the antrum communicates with the mastoid air cells via several openings. The antrum and air cells are lined by mucosa. Anteroinferiorly the antrum is related to the canal for the facial nerve.

Auditory tube

This connects the tympanic cavity to the nasopharynx. The posterior third is bony and the remainder is cartilaginous. The mucosa is continuous with that of the tympanic cavity and nasopharynx.

It equalizes pressure in the middle ear with atmospheric pressure, allowing free movement of the tympanic membrane. Pressure changes, e.g. during flying, can be equalized by swallowing or chewing—these movements open the auditory tubes.

Nerve supply is from the tympanic plexus formed by the facial and glossopharyngeal nerves and from the pterygopalatine ganglion.

Ossicles

These are the incus, malleus, and stapes. The malleus is attached to the tympanic membrane. The incus connects the malleus to the stapes, which is attached to the oval window (Fig. 7.41).

The ossicles transmit vibration from the tympanic membrane to the oval window.

There are two muscles associated with the ossicles:
- Tensor tympani dampens vibration of the tympanic membrane.
- Stapedius dampens vibration of the stapes.

They are innervated by V_3 and VII cranial nerves, respectively.

Walls of the middle ear	
Wall	**Components**
roof (tegmental wall)	tegmen tympani (thin plate of bone): separates cavity from dura in floor of middle cranial fossa
floor (jugular wall)	a layer of bone separates tympanic cavity from superior bulb of internal jugular vein
lateral wall (membranous)	tympanic membrane with epitympanic recess superiorly
medial wall (labyrinthine)	separates tympanic cavity from inner ear
anterior wall (carotid)	separates tympanic cavity from carotid canal; superiorly lies opening of auditory tube and canal for tensor tympani
posterior wall	connected by aditus to mastoid antrum and air cells

Fig. 7.40 Walls of the middle ear.

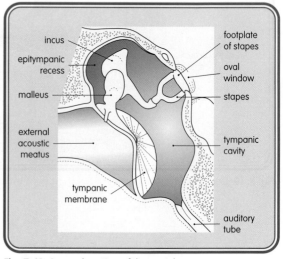

Fig. 7.41 Coronal section of the ossicles.

Internal ear

This lies in the petrous temporal bone (Fig. 7.42). It consists of a bony labyrinth and a membranous labyrinth. The two are separated by a space containing fluid called perilymph.

Bony labyrinth

Cochlea

This contains the cochlear ducts and is concerned with hearing. It makes 2.5 turns about a bony core, the modiolus. The large basal turn of the cochlea produces the promontory on the medial wall of the tympanic cavity.

Vestibule

The vestibule contains the utricle and saccule, components of the balance system. It is continuous with the cochlea anteriorly, with the semicircular canals posteriorly, and with the posterior cranial fossa by the aqueduct of the vestibule. The aqueduct extends to the posterior surface of the petrous temporal bone to open into the internal auditory meatus. It contains the endolymphatic ducts and blood vessels.

Semicircular canals

These communicate with the vestibule and are perpendicular to each other. At one end of each canal is a swelling, the ampulla. The semicircular ducts lie in the canals.

Membranous labyrinth

This is a series of ducts and sacs in the vestibule of the bony labyrinth which contain endolymph.

Cochlear duct

This accommodates the spiral organ (of Corti), which contains the receptors of the auditory apparatus. The spiral organ lies between the scala vestibuli and the scala tympani, both of which are filled with perilymph and which communicate with each other at the tip of the cochlea.

Saccule and utricle

These contain receptors that respond to linear acceleration and the static pull of gravity.

Semicircular ducts

These contain receptors that respond to rotational acceleration in three different planes.

Endolymphatic duct

This duct opens into the endolymphatic sac. Endolymph has a similar composition to intracellular fluid.

Vestibulocochlear nerve (VIII)

Near the lateral end of the internal auditory meatus, the VIII nerve divides into an anterior cochlear nerve (hearing) and a posterior vestibular nerve (balance), as

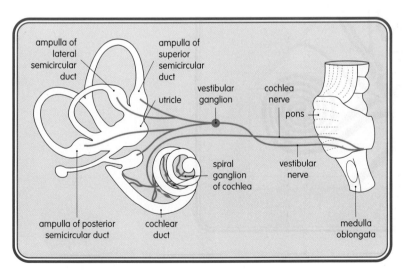

Fig. 7.43 Vestibulocochlear nerve.

shown in Fig. 7.43. The vestibular nerve enlarges to form the vestibular ganglion, and its fibres supply receptors in the semicircular ducts, the saccule, and the utricle. The cochlear nerve forms the spiral ganglion and supplies the spiral organ.

Facial nerve in the temporal bone

The facial nerve (VII) and its sensory root, the nervus intermedius, enter the internal auditory meatus together with the VIII nerve. The two roots fuse and enter the facial canal to pass above the internal ear to reach the medial wall of the middle ear. The nerve then turns sharply above the promontory and passes downwards in the aditus and antrum to leave the temporal bone through the stylomastoid foramen. The sensory geniculate ganglion lies at the sharp bend that the nerve makes on entering the middle ear.

Branches in the temporal bone

These comprise:

- The greater petrosal nerve. This branches off at the geniculate ganglion and enters the middle cranial fossa. It is joined by the deep petrosal nerve to form the nerve of the pterygoid canal.

- The nerve to stapedius.
- The chorda tympani. This is given off just above the stylomastoid foramen. It passes to the posterior wall of the middle ear, crosses the deep surface of the tympanic membrane, and enters a canal leading to the petrotympanic fissure. It joins the lingual nerve in the infratemporal fossa.

○ **Describe the anatomy of the external, middle, and internal ear.**
○ **Discuss the anatomy of the facial nerve in the temporal bone.**

Fig. 7.42 Internal ear.

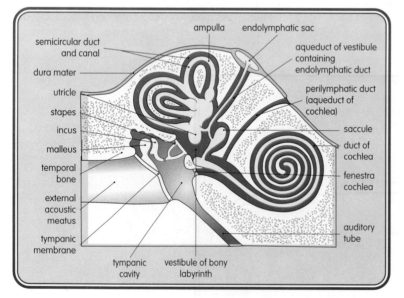

THE SOFT TISSUES OF THE NECK

The neck is the region between the head and the thorax.

Fascial layers of the neck

These are illustrated in Fig. 7.44.

Superficial fascia

This is a thin layer that encloses the platysma muscle. The cutaneous nerves, superficial vessels, and superficial lymph nodes lie in the fascia.

Deep fascia

The deep fascia lies beneath the superficial fascia. It is condensed in certain regions to form the investing layer of deep cervical fascia, the pretracheal fascia, the prevertebral fascia, and the carotid sheath.

Investing layer of deep cervical fascia

This completely encircles the neck, splitting to enclose the sternomastoid and trapezius muscles. Posteriorly it is attached to the ligamentum nuchae. Superiorly it is attached to the hyoid bone. Above this it splits to enclose the submandibular gland and then attaches to the lower border of the mandible. The fascia also splits to enclose the parotid gland and is attached to the zygomatic arch and the base of the skull. The stylomandibular ligament is a thickening of the fascia between the angle of the mandible and the styloid process.

Inferiorly the fascia is attached to the acromion, the clavicle, and the manubrium. It attaches to the anterior and posterior borders of the manubrium to form the suprasternal space, which contains the jugular arch.

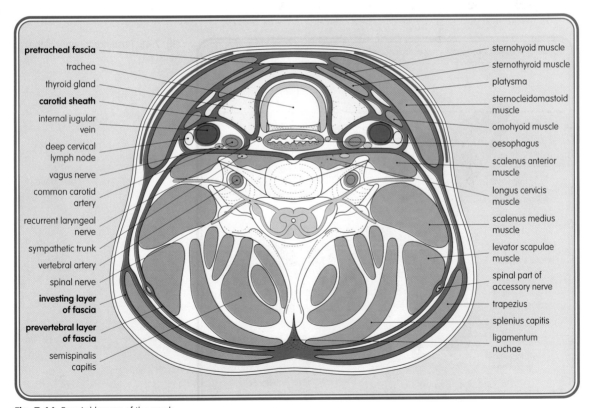

Fig. 7.44 Fascial layers of the neck.

Pretracheal fascia

This is attached superiorly to the thyroid and cricoid cartilages. Inferiorly it enters the thorax to blend with the fibrous pericardium. Laterally it blends with the carotid sheath. It encloses the thyroid gland and the parathyroid glands and lies deep to the infrahyoid muscles.

Prevertebral fascia

This fascia covers the prevertebral muscles (longus capitis, longus colli) and is attached posteriorly to the ligamentum nuchae. It forms the floor of the posterior triangle. Laterally it forms the axillary sheath, which surrounds the axillary artery and the brachial plexus. Superiorly it is attached to the base of the skull and inferiorly it enters the thorax to blend with the anterior longitudinal ligament of the vertebral column. The retropharyngeal space lies between the prevertebral fascia and the pharynx.

Carotid sheath

This is a condensation of the fascia surrounding the common and internal carotid arteries, the internal jugular vein, the deep cervical chain of nodes, and the vagus nerve. It extends from the base of the skull to the root of the neck.

Posterior triangle of the neck

The inferior belly of omohyoid divides the posterior triangle into a large occipital triangle and a small supraclavicular triangle (Fig. 7.45).

The margins and contents of the posterior triangle are detailed in Figs 7.46 and 7.47, respectively.

Fig. 7.48 outlines the muscles on the lateral aspect of the neck.

Cervical plexus

The cervical plexus is formed by the anterior rami of C1–C4 spinal nerves and lies at the origin of levator

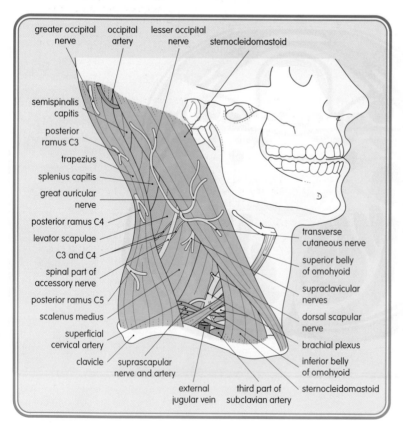

Fig. 7.45 Posterior triangle of the neck.

scapulae and scalenus medius muscles (Fig. 7.49). It is covered by the prevertebral fascia and is related to the internal jugular vein in the carotid sheath.

External jugular vein

This is formed by the union of the posterior auricular vein and the posterior division of the retromandibular vein behind the angle of the mandible. It crosses the sternomastoid and pierces the deep fascia just above

the clavicle in the posterior triangle to enter the subclavian vein.

Contents of the posterior triangle	
Structure	**Origin**
third part of subclavian artery	enters anterior inferior angle of triangle
superficial cervical artery	branch of thyrocervical trunk of subclavian artery
suprascapular artery	branch of thyrocervical trunk
brachial plexus	roots of plexus enter posterior triangle by emerging between scalenus anterior and medius; trunks and cords also lie in posterior triangle before entering the axilla
accessory nerve	spinal part of accessory nerve enters posterior triangle by emerging from deep to posterior border of sternomastoid
cervical plexus	the four cutaneous branches emerge from posterior border of sternomastoid

Fig. 7.47 Contents of the posterior triangle.

Margins of the posterior triangle	
Margin	**Components**
anterior	posterior border of sternomastoid
posterior	anterior border of trapezius
inferior	middle third of clavicle
roof	skin, superficial fascia, platysma, investing layer of deep fascia
floor	prevertebral fascia covering muscles of floor

Fig. 7.46 Margins of the posterior triangle.

Major muscles of the lateral aspect of the neck			
Name of muscle (nerve supply)	**Origin**	**Insertion**	**Action**
platysma (VII nerve)	inferior border of mandible; skin and subcutaneous tisses of lower part of the face	fascia covering superior parts of pectoralis major and deltoid muscles	used to express sadness and fright by pulling angles of mouth down
sternocleidomastoid [XI nerve (spinal part), C2, C3]	anterior surface of manubrium of sternum; medial third of clavicle	mastoid process of temporal bone and superior nuchal line	individually each muscle laterally flexes neck and rotates it so face is turned upwards toward opposite side; both muscles act together to flex neck
trapezius [XI nerve (spinal part), C2, C3]	superior nuchal line; external occipital protuberance; ligamentum nuchae; spinous processes of C7–T12 vertebrae	lateral third of clavicle; acromion; spine of scapula	elevates, retracts, and rotates scapula

Fig. 7.48 Major muscles of the lateral aspect of the neck.

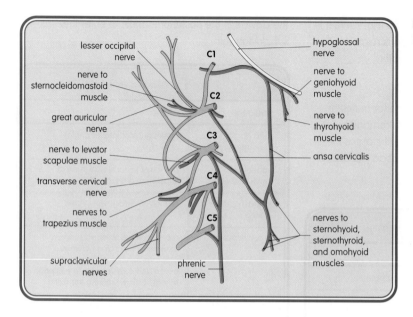

Fig. 7.49 Branches of the cervical plexus.

Anterior triangle of the neck

The anterior triangle is formed by the anterior border of sternocleidomastoid muscle, the midline of the neck, and the inferior border of the mandible. It is subdivided by the anterior and posterior belly of digastric and the superior belly of omohyoid into the digastric (submandibular), carotid, and muscular triangles (Figs 7.50 and 7.51).

The muscles of the anterior triangle are shown in Fig. 7.52, and the contents are detailed in Figs 7.50 and 7.51).

Vessels of the anterior triangle
Common carotid artery

The left common carotid artery arises from the aortic arch, the right from the brachiocephalic trunk. Both ascend in the neck deep to sternomastoid behind the sternoclavicular joint. At the level of the upper border of the thyroid cartilage the arteries divide into the external and internal carotid arteries (Fig. 7.53).

At the terminal part of the common carotid artery and the origin of the internal carotid artery there is a localized dilatation, the carotid sinus. The sinus contains baroreceptors that respond to changes in arterial pressure.

Contents of the anterior triangle of the neck	
Triangle	**Main contents**
carotid	external carotid artery; larynx and pharynx, and internal and external laryngeal nerves
muscular	sternothyroid and sternohyoid muscles, superior belly of omohyoid; thyroid gland, trachea, and oesophagus
digastric (submandibular)	submandibular gland and lymph nodes; facial artery and vein; external carotid artery; internal carotid artery, internal jugular vein, glossopharyngeal (IX), vagus (X), and hypoglossal (XII) nerves
submental	submental lymph nodes

Fig. 7.50 Contents of the anterior triangle of the neck.

The carotid body is embedded in the tunica adventitia of the artery. It contains chemoreceptors that monitor blood carbon dioxide levels.

Both the carotid sinus and the carotid body are innervated by the carotid sinus branch of the IX nerve.

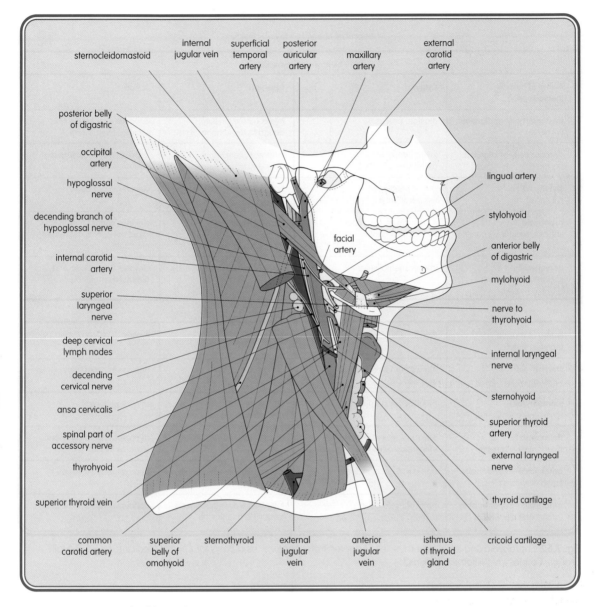

Fig. 7.51 Anterior triangle of the neck.

sternocleidomastoid

internal jugular vein

superficial temporal artery

posterior auricular artery

maxillary artery

external carotid artery

posterior belly of digastric

occipital artery

hypoglossal nerve

decending branch of hypoglossal nerve

internal carotid artery

superior laryngeal nerve

deep cervical lymph nodes

decending cervical nerve

ansa cervicalis

spinal part of accessory nerve

thyrohyoid

superior thyroid vein

common carotid artery

superior belly of omohyoid

sternothyroid

external jugular vein

anterior jugular vein

isthmus of thyroid gland

cricoid cartilage

lingual artery

stylohyoid

facial artery

anterior belly of digastric

mylohyoid

nerve to thyrohyoid

internal laryngeal nerve

sternohyoid

superior thyroid artery

external laryngeal nerve

thyroid cartilage

Suprahyoid and infrahyoid muscles			
Suprahyoid muscles			
Name of muscle (nerve supply)	**Origin**	**Insertion**	**Action**
posterior belly of digastric (VII nerve)	mastoid process	intermediate tendon bound to hyoid bone	depresses mandible and elevates hyoid bone
anterior belly of digastric (V_3 nerve)	lower border of mandible near midline	intermediate tendon bound to hyoid bone	depresses mandible and elevates hyoid bone
stylohyoid (VII nerve)	styloid process of temporal bone	body of hyoid bone	elevates hyoid bone
mylohyoid (inferior alveolar V_3 nerve)	mylohyoid line on medial surface of mandible	body of hyoid bone	elevates floor of mouth and hyoid bone, and depresses mandible
geniohyoid (C1 through XII nerve)	inferior mental spine	body of hyoid bone	elevates hyoid bone and depresses mandible
Infrahyoid muscles			
Name of muscle (nerve supply)	**Origin**	**Insertion**	**Action**
sternohyoid (ansa cervicalis C1–C3)	manubrium sterni and clavicle	body of hyoid bone	depresses hyoid bone
sternothyroid (ansa cervicalis C1–C3)	manubrium sterni	oblique line on lamina of thyroid cartilage	depresses larynx
thyrohyoid (C1 through XII nerve)	oblique line on lamina of thyroid cartilage	body of hyoid bone	depresses hyoid bone and elevates larynx
omohyoid—inferior belly (ansa cervicalis C1–C3)	upper margin of scapula	intermediate tendon bound to clavicle and first rib	depresses hyoid bone
omohyoid—superior belly (ansa cervicalis C1–C3)	body of hyoid bone	intermediate tendon bound to clavicle and first rib	depresses hyoid bone

Fig. 7.52 Suprahyoid and infrahyoid muscles. (Adapted from *Anatomy as a Basis for Clinical Medicine,* by E.C.B. Hall-Craggs. Courtesy of Williams & Wilkins.)

External carotid artery

This commences at the upper border of the thyroid cartilage and ascends to enter the parotid. Its branches comprise the following arteries:

- Ascending pharyngeal.
- Superior thyroid.
- Lingual.
- Facial.
- Posterior auricular.
- Occipital.
- Superficial temporal.
- Maxillary.

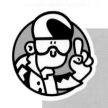

For branches of the external carotid artery use the following mnemonic: **As She Lay Flat Peter Opened Tara's Mouth.**

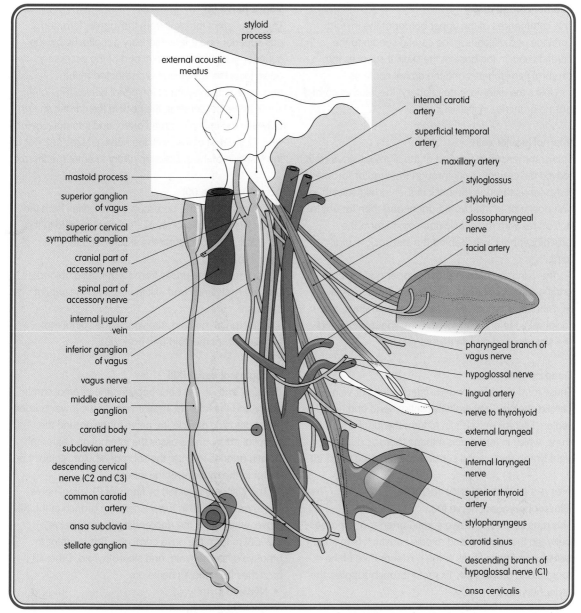

Fig. 7.53 The common carotid artery and the lower cranial nerves. (Adapted from *Clinical Anatomy, An Illustrated Review with Questions and Explanations 2e*, by R.S. Snell. Courtesy of Churchill Livingstone.)

Internal carotid artery

This commences at the upper border of the thyroid cartilage and ascends in the carotid sheath to the carotid canal in the base of the skull. It supplies the cerebral hemispheres and the orbital contents.

Unlike the external carotid artery, the internal carotid has no branches in the neck.

Internal jugular vein

This commences at the end of the sigmoid sinus and leaves the cranial cavity through the jugular foramen. It descends through the neck in the carotid sheath, at first posterior to the carotid artery and then lateral to it. It unites with the subclavian vein to form the brachiocephalic vein behind the sternoclavicular joint.

The vein has dilatations at its upper and lower ends—the superior and inferior bulbs, respectively.

Tributaries include the inferior petrosal sinus, the facial vein, the pharyngeal vein, the lingual vein, and the superior and middle thyroid veins.

Deep cervical nodes

These form a chain along the internal jugular vein in the carotid sheath. They drain the entire head and neck region. Efferent vessels join to form the jugular lymph trunk, which in turn drains into the thoracic duct, the right lymph duct, or the subclavian trunk (see Fig. 7.15).

Nerves of the anterior triangle

Glossopharyngeal nerve (IX)

This runs between the two carotid arteries and passes between the superior and middle constrictors to supply sensory and taste fibres to the posterior third of the tongue and oropharynx. Its motor branch supplies the stylopharyngeus muscle.

Vagus nerve (X)

The vagus exits the skull from the jugular foramen. It has superior and inferior sensory ganglia. Below the superior ganglion the cranial part of the accessory nerve joins the vagus and is distributed to the pharyngeal and recurrent laryngeal nerves (Fig. 7.54). The X nerve descends in the neck in the carotid sheath between the internal carotid artery and internal jugular vein. At the root of the neck the nerve passes anterior to the first part of the subclavian artery to enter the thorax.

Accessory nerve (XI)

The spinal part of the accessory nerve arises from the upper five cervical segments. The roots ascend in the vertebral canal and enter the skull via the foramen magnum.

The cranial root arises from the medulla oblongata. The two roots unite and exit the skull via the jugular foramen.

The cranial root joins the vagus; the spinal root supplies sternomastoid and trapezius.

Hypoglossal nerve (XII)

This descends in the neck between the internal carotid artery and the internal jugular vein. At the lower border of the digastric muscle the nerve loops around the occipital artery and crosses the internal and external carotid arteries to enter the submandibular region. It is motor to the muscles of the tongue.

The XII nerve is joined by fibres of C1 spinal nerve. These are given off in the descending branch of the XII nerve, which joins the descending cervical nerve (C2–C3) to form the ansa cervicalis. This is motor to omohyoid, sternohyoid, and sternothyroid. Other C1 branches from the XII nerve are:

- Nerve to thyrohyoid.
- Nerve to geniohyoid.

Sympathetic trunk

The trunk lies deep in the neck, between the carotid sheath and prevertebral fascia. It has superior, middle, and inferior ganglia. The inferior ganglion usually fuses with the first thoracic ganglion to form the stellate ganglion. Postganglionic fibres form plexuses around the major vessels and supply the structures of the head and neck, e.g. blood vessels and glands, and also give off cardiac branches.

- Describe the deep fascia of the neck.
- Discuss the posterior and anterior triangles of the neck and their contents.

Branches of the vagus nerve	
Branch	**Course and distribution**
meningeal branch	dura mater of posterior cranial fossa
auricular branch	medial surface of auricle, external auditory meatus, and adjacent tympanic membrane
pharyngeal branch	contains motor fibres from XI nerve (cranial part); combines with pharyngeal branches of IX nerve (sensory fibres) to form pharyngeal plexus, which supplies all pharyngeal muscles except stylopharyngeus (IX) and all soft-palate muscles except tensor palatini (V$_3$)
superior laryngeal nerve divides into internal and external laryngeal nerves	internal laryngeal nerve is sensory to piriform fossa and mucosa of larynx above vocal folds; external laryngeal nerve is motor to cricothyroid muscle
cardiac branches	assist in forming cardiac plexus in thorax
right recurrent laryngeal nerve	arises from X nerve as it crosses subclavian artery; hooks backwards and upwards behind artery and ascends in a groove between trachea and oesophagus; supplies all laryngeal muscles (except cricothyroid) and laryngeal mucosa below vocal folds
left recurrent laryngeal nerve	arises from X nerve as it crosses aortic arch; hooks beneath arch behind ligamentum arteriosum and passes into neck between trachea and oesophagus; has a similar distribution to right nerve

Fig. 7.54 Branches of the vagus nerve.

MIDLINE STRUCTURES OF THE FACE AND NECK

Pharynx

The pharynx is a fibromuscular tube lying behind the nasal cavity (nasopharynx), the oral cavity (oropharynx), and the larynx (laryngopharynx). It extends from the base of the skull to the inferior border of the cricoid cartilage (C6 vertebra level), where it is continuous with the oesophagus. There are three layers in the pharyngeal wall:

- The muscular layer is formed by the pharyngeal constrictors and longitudinal muscles (Figs 7.55 and 7.56).
- The pharyngobasilar fascia separates the mucosa and the muscle layer. It blends with the periosteum of the base of the skull.
- The mucous membrane (Fig. 7.57).

Nasopharynx

The nasopharynx lies behind the nasal cavity above the soft palate. During swallowing the soft palate elevates and the pharyngeal wall is pulled forward to form a seal, preventing food entering the nasopharynx. The pharyngeal tonsil lies in the posterior wall. Tubal elevations in the lateral wall are the sites of opening of the auditory tube. The tubal recess is a small depression in the lateral wall, behind the tubal elevation.

Oropharynx

The oropharynx extends from the soft palate to the upper border of the epiglottis. The palatine tonsils lie in its lateral walls. The posterior third of the tongue forms the anterior wall of the oropharynx. It has an irregular surface owing to the presence of the underlying lingual tonsils.

The mucosa is reflected from the tongue onto the epiglottis to form a median and two lateral glossoepiglottic folds. The depression on each side of the median fold is the vallecula.

Laryngopharynx

The laryngopharynx lies behind the laryngeal opening and the posterior surface of the larynx.

The piriform fossa is a groove on either side of the laryngeal inlet. It leads from the back of the tongue to the oesophagus.

Vessels of the pharynx

Blood supply is from branches of the ascending

Muscles of the pharynx			
Name of muscle (nerve supply)	**Origin**	**Insertion**	**Action**
superior constrictor (pharyngeal plexus)	medial pterygoid plate, pterygoid hamulus, pterygomandibular ligament, mylohyoid line of mandible	pharyngeal tubercle of occipital bone, midline raphe	assists in separating oro- and nasopharynx and propels food bolus downward
middle constrictor (pharyngeal plexus)	stylohyoid ligament, lesser and greater cornua of hyoid bone	pharyngeal raphe	propels food bolus downward
inferior constrictor (pharyngeal plexus)	lamina of thyroid cartilage, cricoid cartilage	pharyngeal raphe	propels food bolus downward
cricopharyngeus (pharyngeal plexus)	fibres of inferior constrictor muscle attached to cricoid cartilage	pharyngeal raphe	sphincter at lower end of pharynx
palatopharyngeus (pharyngeal plexus)	palatine aponeurosis	thyroid cartilage	elevates pharyngeal wall and pulls palatopharyngeal folds medially
salpingopharyngeus (pharyngeal plexus)	auditory tube	merges with palatopharyngeus	elevates pharynx and larynx
stylopharyngeus (IX)	styloid process of temporal bone	thyroid cartilage	elevates larynx during swallowing

Fig. 7.55 Muscles of the pharynx.

Fig. 7.56 Muscles of the pharynx.

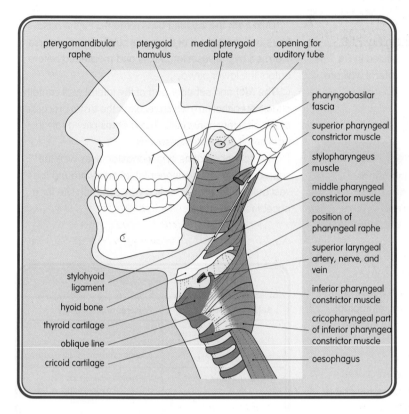

pterygomandibular raphe
pterygoid hamulus
medial pterygoid plate
opening for auditory tube
pharyngobasilar fascia
superior pharyngeal constrictor muscle
stylopharyngeus muscle
middle pharyngeal constrictor muscle
position of pharyngeal raphe
superior laryngeal artery, nerve, and vein
inferior pharyngeal constrictor muscle
cricopharyngeal part of inferior pharyngeal constrictor muscle
oesophagus
stylohyoid ligament
hyoid bone
thyroid cartilage
oblique line
cricoid cartilage

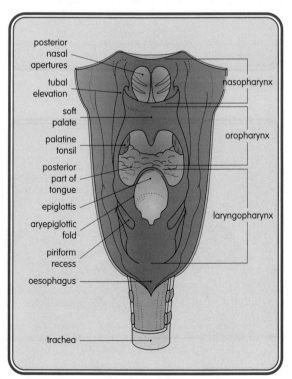

posterior nasal apertures
tubal elevation
soft palate
palatine tonsil
posterior part of tongue
epiglottis
aryepiglottic fold
piriform recess
oesophagus
trachea
nasopharynx
oropharynx
laryngopharynx

Fig. 7.57 Mucous membrane and the interior of the pharynx.

pharyngeal, ascending palatine, facial, maxillary, and lingual arteries.

Veins drain via the pharyngeal venous plexus to the internal jugular vein.

Lymphatics drain into the deep cervical nodes either directly or indirectly via the retropharyngeal or paratracheal nodes.

Nerve supply of the pharynx

This is as follows:

- Motor: cranial part of XI via the pharyngeal plexus.
- Sensory: nasopharynx—maxillary nerve (V_2); oropharynx—IX nerve; laryngopharynx—internal laryngeal nerve (X).

Nose

This consists of:

- The external nose—this has a bony (nasal bones, frontal process of the maxilla) and cartilaginous skeleton, separated by the nasal septum.
- The nasal cavities—these communicate with the external nose via the nares or nostrils, and with the nasopharynx via the choanae.

165

Nasal cavity

The walls of the nasal cavity are listed in Fig. 7.58.

The openings in the lateral wall are listed in Fig 7.59.

The nerve and blood supply of the lateral wall are illustrated in Fig. 7.60.

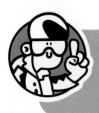

The nasal septum and the external nose both have cartilaginous and bony components.

Paranasal sinuses

These lie around the nasal cavity, in the bones of the face and skull. They are the sphenoidal, ethmoidal, frontal, and maxillary sinuses. They drain into the nasal cavity.

Mucous membrane of the nose

The vestibule lies just inside the anterior nares and is lined by hairy skin. The remainder of the nasal cavity is lined by ciliated columnar epithelium. There is a rich vascular plexus in the submucosa, together with numerous serous and mucous glands.

Dust from the inspired air is removed by the nasal hairs and the mucus of the nasal cavity. The air is also warmed by the vascular plexus and moistened before it enters the lower airway.

The roof and superior part of the lateral wall contains olfactory epithelium, which receives the distal processes of the olfactory nerve cells. These fibres play a role in both smell and taste sensations.

The sphenopalatine artery anastomoses with the septal branch of the superior labial artery around the vestibule of the nose. This is a very common site for a nosebleed (epistaxis).

Openings in the lateral wall of the nose	
Region of lateral wall	**Features and openings**
sphenoethmoidal recess	sphenoidal sinus
superior meatus	posterior ethmoidal air sinuses
middle meatus	the hiatus semilunaris lies below the middle concha; the frontal sinus, anterior ethmoidal, and maxillary sinus open into the hiatus; the bulla ethmoidalis is formed by the underlying middle ethmoidal sinus which opens onto it
inferior meatus	nasolacrimal duct

Fig. 7.59 Openings in the lateral wall of the nose.

Walls of the nasal cavity	
Surface	**Components**
floor	palatine process of maxilla, horizontal process of palatine bone—i.e. the hard palate
roof	nasal, frontal, sphenoid, and ethmoid bones; above lies the anterior cranial fossa and the sphenoidal sinus
lateral wall	maxillary, palatine, sphenoid, lacrimal, and ethmoid bones and the inferior concha; the superior and middle conchae are projections of the ethmoid bone; the three conchae divide the lateral wall into the superior, middle, and inferior meatus and the sphenoethmoidal recess; the last lies above the superior concha
medial wall (nasal septum)	the perpendicular plate of the septal cartilage, the vomer, and the ethmoid

Fig. 7.58 Walls of the nasal cavity.

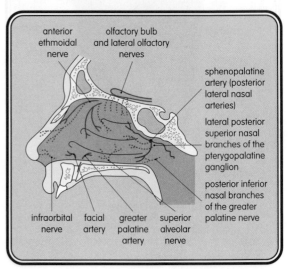

Fig. 7.60 Nerve and blood supply of the lateral wall of the nose.

Pterygopalatine fossa

This is a small pyramidal space lying inferior to the apex of the orbit. It contains the terminal branches of the maxillary artery, the maxillary nerve, the nerve of the pterygoid canal, and the pterygopalatine ganglion. The communications of the fossa are listed in Fig. 7.61.

Communications of the pterygopalatine fossa	
Surface	Communicates with
lateral	infratemporal fossa
medial	nasal cavity via the sphenopalatine foramen
anterior	orbit via the inferior orbital fissure
posterosuperior	middle cranial fossa via the foramen rotundum and pterygoid canal

Fig. 7.61 Communications of the pterygopalatine fossa.

Pterygopalatine ganglion

This is a parasympathetic ganglion lying in the pterygopalatine fossa, just lateral to the sphenopalatine foramen.

Preganglionic fibres from the superior salivary nucleus of the VII nerve enter the greater petrosal nerve. This joins the deep petrosal (sympathetic) nerve to form the nerve of the pterygoid canal, which joins the ganglion. Here the parasympathetic fibres synapse and sympathetic fibres pass uninterrupted through the ganglion. Fibres of common sensation enter the ganglion via ganglionic branches of the maxillary nerve.

The branches of the ganglion are shown in Fig. 7.62.

Oral cavity

This is divided into the vestibule and the oral cavity proper:

- The vestibule lies between the lips and cheeks externally and between the gums and teeth internally.
- The oral cavity proper is bounded by the teeth and gums anteriorly and laterally. The palate forms the roof; the floor is formed by the anterior two-thirds of the tongue. A midline fold of mucosa, the frenulum, lies beneath the tongue (Fig. 7.63).

The submandibular ducts open onto the submandibular papilla on either side of the frenulum. The sublingual fold extends back from the papilla and overlies the sublingual glands. There are also numerous minor salivary glands that open in the oral cavity.

Branches of the pterygopalatine ganglion	
Branch	Course and distribution
nasopalatine nerve	passes through the sphenopalatine foramen to supply the nasal septum and incisive gum of the hard palate
lateral posterior superior nasal nerve	exits via the sphenopalatine foramen to supply the lateral wall of the nose
greater palatine nerve	passes through the greater palatine canal and foramen to supply the mucosa of the palate and the lateral wall of the nose
lesser palatine nerve	exits through the lesser palatine foramina to supply the soft palate and the mucosa over the palatine tonsil
pharyngeal nerve	passes via the palatovaginal canal to supply the nasopharynx
lacrimal fibres	parasympathetic fibres to the lacrimal gland

Fig. 7.62 Branches of the pterygopalatine ganglion.

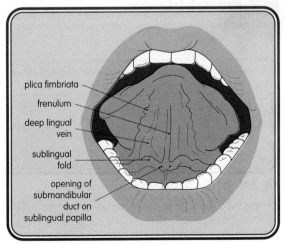

plica fimbriata
frenulum
deep lingual vein
sublingual fold
opening of submandibular duct on sublingual papilla

Fig. 7.63 Oral cavity.

Nerve supply is as follows:
- Roof—greater palatine and nasopalatine nerves.
- Floor—lingual nerve.
- Cheek—buccal nerve (from V_3 nerve).

Lips

The two lips seal the oral cavity anteriorly and also assist in speech. The lips are covered by mucosa internally and by skin externally. The orbicularis oris muscle, the superior and inferior labial vessels and nerves, and numerous minor salivary glands lie in the substance of the lips.

Tongue

This is a mobile muscular organ covered by mucous membrane. The anterior two-thirds lie in the mouth, the posterior third in the oropharynx (Fig. 7.64).

The muscles of the tongue are listed in Fig. 7.65.

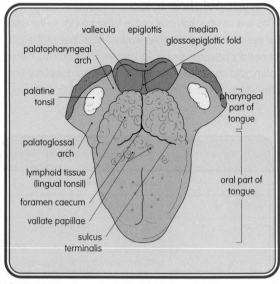

Fig. 7.64 Tongue.

Muscles of the tongue			
Intrinsic muscles			
Name of muscle (nerve supply)	Origin	Insertion	Action
longitudinal (XII nerve)	mucous membrane	mucous membrane	shortens tongue
transverse (XII nerve)	mucous membrane	mucous membrane	narrows tongue
vertical (XII nerve)	median septum and submucosa	mucous membrane	lowers tongue
Extrinsic muscles			
Name of muscle (nerve supply)	Origin	Insertion	Action
palatoglossus (pharyngeal plexus)	palatine aponeurosis	lateral aspect of tongue	pulls tongue upward and backward and narrows oropharyngeal isthmus
genioglossus (XII nerve)	superior mental genial spine of mandible	merges with other tongue muscles	draws tongue forward and pulls tip backward
hyoglossus (XII nerve)	body and greater cornu of hyoid bone	merges with other tongue muscles	depresses tongue
styloglossus (XII nerve)	styloid process of temporal bone	merges with other tongue muscles	draws tongue upward and backward

Fig. 7.65 Muscles of the tongue.

Mucous membrane of the tongue

The sulcus terminalis divides the tongue into the anterior two-thirds and the posterior third. The foramen caecum lies at the apex of the sulcus. It is the remnant of the upper end of the thyroglossal duct. Between 10 and 12 vallate papillae lie anterior to the sulcus.

The mucosa of the anterior two-thirds of the tongue is relatively smooth and has numerous filiform and fungiform papillae on the dorsal surface. The frenulum connects it to the floor of the mouth. Lateral folds of mucosa, the plica fimbriata, are also seen on the ventral surface of the tongue.

The irregular surface of the posterior third of the tongue is caused by the underlying lingual tonsils.

Blood and nerve supply to the tongue

Vessels of the tongue comprise the lingual arteries and veins.

Lymphatic drainage is to the deep cervical, the submandibular, and the submental nodes. Carcinoma of the tongue may spread via the lymphatics to both sides of the neck, dramatically worsening its prognosis.

The nerve supply to the tongue is shown in Fig. 7.66.

Remember, the XII nerve is motor to all the muscles of the tongue except palatoglossus (pharyngeal plexus).

Floor of the mouth and submandibular region

This region lies between the mandible and hyoid bone. It contains the following:

- Muscles: digastric, mylohyoid, hyoglossus, geniohyoid, genioglossus, and styloglossus.
- Salivary glands: submandibular and sublingual.
- Nerves: lingual, glossopharyngeal, and hypoglossal; submandibular ganglion.
- Blood vessels: facial and lingual.
- Lymph nodes: submandibular.

Submandibular gland

This consists of two parts—a large superficial part and a small deep part—which are continuous around the posterior border of mylohyoid. The deep part of the gland lies between the mylohyoid superficially and the styloglossus and hyoglossus.

Blood supply is from the facial and lingual arteries.

Nerve supply is from the submandibular ganglion, a parasympathetic ganglion with the following features:

- Preganglionic parasympathetic fibres originate in the superior salivary nucleus of the VII nerve and pass to the ganglion via the nervus intermedius, the chorda tympani, and the lingual nerve.
- Sympathetic and sensory fibres from the superior cervical ganglion and the lingual nerve pass through the ganglion.
- Postganglionic parasympathetic secretomotor fibres pass to the submandibular and sublingual glands via the lingual nerve or directly.

Fig. 7.66 Nerve supply to the tongue.

Nerve supply to the tongue		
	Posterior third	**Anterior two-thirds**
general sensory	glossopharyngeal nerve (IX)	lingual nerve (V_3)
taste	glossopharyngeal nerve (IX)	chorda tympani (VII) (via the lingual nerve)
motor	hypoglossal nerve, pharyngeal plexus (palatoglossus) (XII, XI)	hypoglossal nerve (XII)

Lingual nerve

From the mandibular third-molar region, the lingual nerve passes across styloglossus to the lateral surface of hyoglossus and across the submandibular duct, to break up into its terminal branches supplying the mucosa of the tongue.

Hypoglossal nerve

In the submandibular region, the hypoglossal nerve runs forward below the deep part of the submandibular gland, the submandibular duct, and the lingual nerve. It divides into its terminal branches and supplies all the muscles of the tongue except palatoglossus.

Sublingual gland

This gland lies superficially under the mucosa of the floor of the mouth. The lingual nerve and submandibular duct lie medially. It is supplied by the submandibular ganglion.

Palate and tonsils

The palate forms the roof of the mouth and the floor of the nose. It is divided into two components:

• The hard palate is composed of the palatine process of the maxilla and the horizontal process of the palatine bone. It is covered by mucous membrane.
• The soft palate is a mobile fibromuscular fold lying posteriorly. It is composed of muscles (Fig. 7.67) and the palatine aponeurosis—the expanded tendon of tensor veli palatini.

Blood supply to the palate is from the greater and lesser palatine arteries. Nerve supply is from the pterygopalatine ganglion.

The palatine tonsils are masses of lymphoid tissue lying in the tonsillar fossae between the palatoglossal and palatopharyngeal arches. They are covered by mucous membrane. The surface is pitted by many openings that lead to the tonsillar crypts. Lymphatics drain to the deep cervical nodes.

Larynx

The larynx is continuous with the laryngopharynx superiorly and with the trachea inferiorly. It acts as a sphincter, separating the respiratory system from the alimentary system, and is responsible for voice production.

The laryngeal cartilages are shown in Fig. 7.68. The laryngeal membranes link these cartilages together and join the larynx to the hyoid bone and the trachea (Fig. 7.69). The membranes thicken in places to form ligaments.

Mucous membrane of the larynx

The mucosa is tucked under the vestibular ligament to form the laryngeal ventricle between the vestibular and vocal folds. Above the vocal fold the mucosa is supplied by the internal laryngeal nerve and the superior laryngeal artery; below the vocal fold it is supplied by the recurrent laryngeal nerve and the inferior laryngeal artery (from the superior thyroid artery).

Muscles of the soft palate			
Name of muscle (nerve supply)	**Origin**	**Insertion**	**Action**
tensor veli palatini (nerve to medial pterygoid V_3)	spine of sphenoid, auditory tube	with muscle of other side, forms palatine aponeurosis	tenses soft palate
levator veli palatini (pharyngeal plexus)	petrous part of temporal bone, auditory tube	palatine aponeurosis	elevates soft palate
musculus uvulae (pharyngeal plexus)	posterior border of hard palate	mucous membrane of uvula	elevates uvula
palatopharyngeus (pharyngeal plexus)	palatine aponeurosis	posterior border of thyroid cartilage	elevates pharyngeal wall and pulls palatopharyngeal folds medially
palatoglossus (pharyngeal plexus)	palatine aponeurosis	lateral aspect of tongue	pulls tongue upward and backward and narrows oropharyngeal isthmus

Fig. 7.67 Muscles of the soft palate.

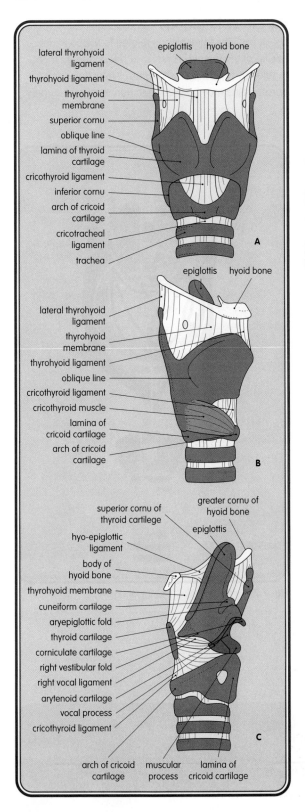

Fig. 7.68 Laryngeal cartilages from the front (A), from the lateral aspect (B), and without the left lamina of thyroid cartilage (C).

Laryngeal membranes	
Membrane	**Attachments**
thyrohyoid	runs between the thyroid cartilage and hyoid bone; has a midline thickening and two lateral thickenings, the median ligament and lateral thyrohyoid ligaments, respectively
quadrangular	runs between the epiglottis and the arytenoid cartilage; its lower free border is the vestibular ligament
cricothyroid	joins the cricoid, thyroid, and arytenoid cartilages; its upper free border is the vocal ligament; there is also a midline thickening, the median cricothyroid ligament
cricotracheal	runs from the cricoid cartilage to the trachea

Fig. 7.69 Laryngeal membranes.

Laryngeal cavity

The laryngeal inlet allows communication between the pharynx and the larynx. It is bounded by the epiglottis and the aryepiglottic and interarytenoid folds (Fig. 7.70).

The inlet leads to the vestibule, which extends to the vestibular folds. The laryngeal ventricle lies between the vestibular and vocal folds. The rima glottidis is the space between the vocal folds. The infraglottic cavity lies below the vocal folds and is continuous with the trachea.

Trachea

The trachea commences at the level of C6 vertebra and is continuous with the larynx above. It ends at the sternal angle by dividing into the right and left main bronchi. Its walls are reinforced by C-shaped hyaline cartilage anteriorly.

Thyroid gland

This endocrine organ, lying anteriorly in the neck, has two lobes connected by a narrow isthmus (Fig. 7.71). It regulates the metabolic rate by producing the hormone thyroxine.

Parathyroid glands

These are four small glands related to the posterior border of the thyroid gland. They are important in the regulation of calcium metabolism. Note, the parathyroids may be damaged during thyroid surgery.

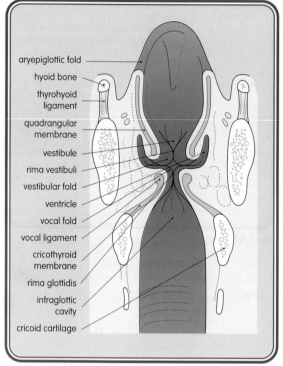

Fig. 7.70 Coronal section of the laryngeal cavity.

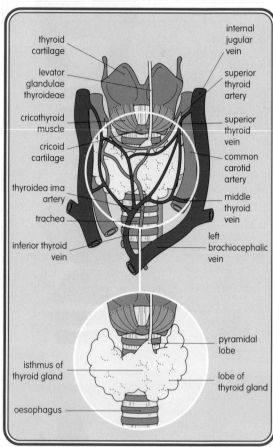

Fig. 7.71 Anterior view of the thyroid gland.

- Describe the anatomy of the pharynx and larynx.
- Outline the anatomy of the oral cavity and its contents, including the tongue, palate, and tonsils.
- Describe the anatomy of the submandibular region.
- Summarize the anatomy of the thyroid gland.

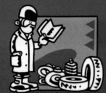

8. The Back

REGIONS AND COMPONENTS OF THE BACK

The back consists of the vertebral column, the spinal cord and the roots of the spinal nerves, and associated muscles.

The vertebral column extends from the skull to the coccyx. It supports the weight of the body above the pelvic girdle. There is limited movement between adjacent vertebrae, but the total movement of the entire column is considerable.

There are 33 vertebrae arranged in five regions (seven cervical, 12 thoracic, five lumbar, five sacral, and four coccygeal). The sacral and coccygeal vertebrae fuse to form the sacrum and coccyx, respectively (see Fig. 8.2).

There are four curvatures of the vertebral column in adults. The cervical and lumbar curvatures (secondary curvatures) are concave posteriorly; the thoracic and sacrococcygeal curvatures (primary curvatures) are concave anteriorly. The primary curvatures develop during the foetal period, whereas the secondary curvatures begin to appear before birth but become obvious only during infancy.

SURFACE ANATOMY AND SUPERFICIAL STRUCTURES

Visible and palpable features of the back are shown in Fig. 8.1. Note the following:
- The first palpable spine when passing a finger down the back of the neck is that of C7.
- The inferior angle of the scapula lies at the angle of the spine of T7 vertebra.
- A line passing through the highest point of the iliac crest passes through the spine of L4 vertebra.

Cutaneous innervation of the back
The skin and muscles of the back are supplied segmentally by the posterior rami of the 31 pairs of spinal nerves. The posterior rami of the 1st, 6th, 7th, and 8th cervical nerves and the 4th and 5th lumbar nerves supply the deep muscles of the back and do not supply the skin.

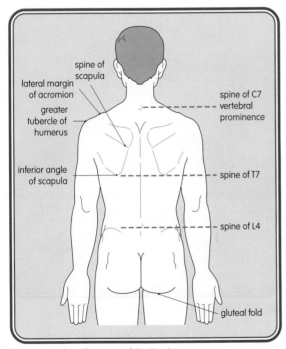

Fig. 8.1 Surface features of the back.

spine of scapula
lateral margin of acromion
greater tubercle of humerus
inferior angle of scapula
spine of C7 vertebral prominence
spine of T7
spine of L4
gluteal fold

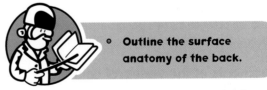

Outline the surface anatomy of the back.

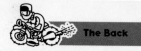

THE VERTEBRAL COLUMN

Skeleton of the vertebral column

The vertebral column consists of 33 vertebrae lying in five regions (Fig. 8.2). Individual vertebrae articulate with each other via intervertebral discs.

The vertebral column supports the weight of the upper body. The weight is transferred to the lower limb via the pelvic girdle. It also transmits and protects the spinal cord.

Features of individual vertebrae

The cervical and thoracic vertebrae, together with the sacrum and coccyx, are discussed in Chapter 4.

Fig. 8.3 illustrates the features of typical lumbar vertebrae.

Joints of the vertebral column

The craniovertebral joints are discussed in Chapter 7.

Intervertebral discs

These are the joints between the bodies of adjacent vertebrae (Fig. 8.4). They are secondary cartilaginous joints. The joints provide strength and weight-bearing capacity, and absorb compressive forces.

The disc is composed of:
- The annulus fibrosus, an outer ring made up of concentric layers of fibrous tissue.
- The nucleus pulposus, a gelatinous core lying close to the posterior border.

Damage to the disc may cause prolapse or herniation of the nucleus pulposus—a slipped disc. This is commonest in the lumbar region.

Joints of the vertebral arches

These are between the articular processes on the vertebral arches. They are plane synovial joints.

Ligaments of the vertebral column

These are described in Fig. 8.5.

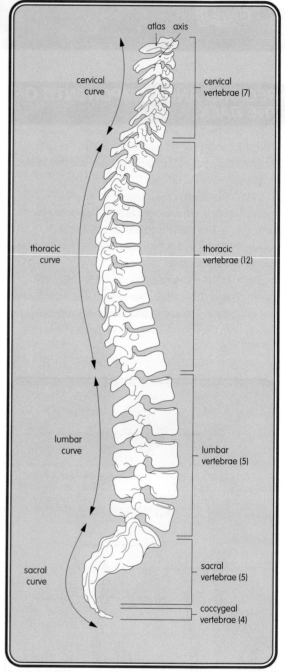

Fig. 8.2 Lateral view of the vertebral column.

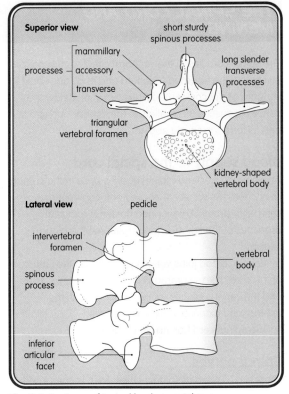

Superior view

processes — mammillary
— accessory
— transverse

short sturdy spinous processes

long slender transverse processes

triangular vertebral foramen

kidney-shaped vertebral body

Lateral view

pedicle

intervertebral foramen

spinous process

vertebral body

inferior articular facet

Fig. 8.3 Features of typical lumbar vertebrae.

intervertebral foramen

spinal nerve

supraspinous ligament

interspinous ligament

ligamentum flavum

posterior longitudinal ligament

body

anterior longitudinal ligament

annulus fibrosus

nucleus pulposus

Fig. 8.4 Sagittal section of vertebrae showing the intercostal discs and ligaments of the vertebral column.

Fig. 8.5 Ligaments of the vertebral column.

Ligaments of the vertebral column	
Ligament	**Action**
anterior longitudinal	strong band covering the anterior part of the vertebral bodies and the intervertebral discs running from the anterior tubercle of C1 vertebra to the sacrum; maintains stability of the intervertebral discs and prevents hyperextension of the vertebral column
posterior longitudinal	is attached to the posterior aspect of the intervertebral discs and posterior edges of the vertebral bodies from C2 vertebra to the sacrum; prevents hyperflexion of the vertebral column and posterior protrusion of the discs
supraspinous	accessory ligament uniting the tips of the spinous processes
interspinous	accessory ligaments uniting the spinous processes
ligamenta flava	help to preserve the curvature of the vertebral column and support the joints between the vertebral arches; unite the laminae of adjacent vertebrae

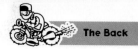
Movement of the vertebral column

Flexion, extension, lateral flexion, and rotation are possible. Mobility results from the compression and elasticity of the intervertebral discs.

Muscles of the vertebral column

There are three main groups of muscles:

- The superficial muscles associated with the upper limb—trapezius, latissimus dorsi, levator scapulae, and rhomboideus minor and major.
- The intermediate muscles—serratus posterior and levatores costarum.
- The deep muscles of the back—superficial vertical running (erector spinae), intermediate oblique running (transversospinalis), and deepest muscles (interspinales and intertransversarii).

Blood supply to the vertebral column

Spinal arteries supplying the vertebral column are branches of:

- Vertebral and ascending cervical arteries of the neck.
- Posterior intercostal arteries in the thoracic region.
- Subcostal and lumbar arteries in the abdomen.
- Iliolumbar and lateral sacral arteries in the sacrum.

Spinal veins form plexuses inside (internal vertebral venous plexus) and outside (external vertebral venous plexus) the vertebral canal.

Blood may return from the pelvis and abdomen to the heart via the vertebral venous plexuses and the superior vena cava. Abdominal and pelvic tumours may metastasize to the vertebrae in this way.

○ **Describe the bones and joints of the vertebral column.**

THE SPINAL CORD AND MENINGES

The spinal cord lies in the vertebral canal. It commences just below the foramen magnum and ends opposite L2 vertebra at the conus medullaris (Fig. 8.6). Below the conus medullaris the rootlets of the lumbar and sacral nerves form the cauda equina.

Blood supply to the spinal cord

Anterior and posterior spinal arteries arise in the cranial cavity from the vertebral arteries or the inferior cerebellar artery. Anterior and posterior radicular branches of the spinal arteries reinforce the blood supply.

Venous blood joins venous plexuses on the surface of the cord. These communicate with the cranial veins and the venous sinuses of the skull and with the internal and external vertebral plexuses.

The spinal cord has no lymphatic vessels.

Spinal nerves

There are 31 pairs of spinal nerves. Each is composed of a dorsal and ventral root (see Fig. 1.9).

Spinal meninges and cerebrospinal fluid (CSF)

The meninges and the CSF surround and protect the spinal cord.

Dura mater

This is tough fibrous membrane continuous with the dura of the brain. It is separated from the vertebral periosteum by the epidural space. It is attached to the foramen magnum superiorly and to the coccyx inferiorly by the filum terminale.

Arachnoid mater

This is a delicate membrane that is separated from the dura by a potential space, the subdural space. Like the dura it covers the spinal nerve roots and spinal ganglia. The subarachnoid space lies between the arachnoid and pia. CSF is present in this space.

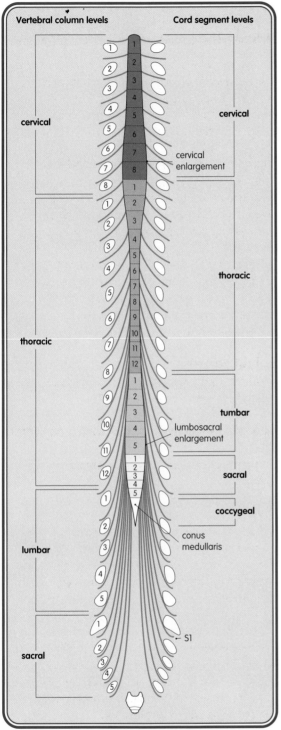

Fig. 8.6 Spinal cord, showing vertebral and segmental levels. (Adapted from *Anatomy as a Basis for Clinical Medicine*, by E.C.B. Hall-Craggs. Courtesy of Williams & Wilkins.)

Pia mater

This is a finely vascular membrane that is closely adherent to the spinal cord. It covers the roots of the spinal nerves and the spinal ganglia. Below the conus medullaris the pia continues as the filum terminale. It pierces the dural sac to attach to the coccyx.

Lumbar puncture

The spinal cord ceases at the level of L2 vertebra, but the meninges continue well below this. By inserting a needle into the subarachnoid space below L2, a sample of CSF may be obtained without damaging the cord.

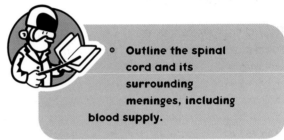

○ **Outline the spinal cord and its surrounding meninges, including blood supply.**

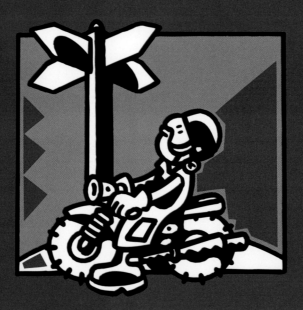

SELF-ASSESSMENT

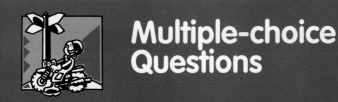

Multiple-choice Questions

Indicate whether each answer is true or false.

1. The diaphragm:

(a) Has a motor nerve supply from the phrenic nerve only.
(b) Transmits the aorta at the level of T10 vertebra.
(c) Transmits the inferior vena cava through the central tendon.
(d) Is pierced by the sympathetic trunks.
(e) Is the main muscle used in quiet expiration.

2. Regarding the heart:

(a) It is completely surrounded by pericardium that is attached to the left dome of the diaphragm.
(b) It has the fossa ovalis lying on the interatrial wall.
(c) It is supplied by coronary arteries that arise from the aortic sinuses.
(d) The sinoatrial node is the normal cardiac pacemaker.
(e) The mitral valve lies in the left atrioventricular orifice.

3. Regarding the thoracic aorta:

(a) The ascending aorta has no branches.
(b) The aortic arch is attached to the right pulmonary artery via the ligamentum arteriosum.
(c) The descending aorta commences opposite the sternal angle.
(d) The descending aorta gives off branches to the pericardium, bronchi, and oesophagus.
(e) The aorta leaves the thorax by passing through the central tendon of the diaphragm at the level of T12 vertebra.

4. Concerning the lungs and bronchi:

(a) The left main bronchus is shorter, wider, and more vertical than the right.
(b) The right lung has three lobes and the left lung has two lobes.
(c) The bronchopulmonary segments are the functional units of the lungs.
(d) The apex of the lung lies below the clavicle.
(e) The visceral pleura has a rich somatic innervation and is very sensitive to pain.

5. Regarding the thoracic wall and the intercostal spaces:

(a) The thoracic wall is made up of both bone and cartilage.
(b) The neurovascular bundle runs deep to the three muscle layers.
(c) The intercostal nerves are the posterior rami of the thoracic spinal nerves.
(d) The motor innervation to the intercostal muscles is from the phrenic nerve and the intercostal nerves.
(e) The intercostal arteries all arise from the aorta.

6. Concerning thoracic nerves:

(a) The phrenic nerves pass anterior to the root of the lungs.
(b) The phrenic nerve arises from the ventral rami of C3–C5 spinal nerves.
(c) The vagus and phrenic nerves contribute to the formation of the pulmonary and oesophageal plexuses.
(d) Both the right and left vagi leave the thorax lying anterior to the oesophagus.
(e) The thoracic sympathetic ganglia are concerned with supplying intrathoracic structures only.

7. Regarding the inguinal canal:

(a) The superficial inguinal ring is an opening in the external oblique aponeurosis.
(b) The deep inguinal ring is a defect in the internal oblique muscle.
(c) The spermatic cord with its three coverings is formed at the deep inguinal ring.
(d) The ilioinguinal nerve enters the inguinal canal via the deep inguinal ring.
(e) The canal lies above and parallel to the inguinal ligament.

8. The stomach:

(a) Is derived from the foregut.
(b) Has a fundus that lies above the level of entry of the oesophagus.
(c) Is not covered by peritoneum over the fundus.
(d) Has a blood supply derived mainly from the coeliac trunk.
(e) Drains mainly into the azygos system of veins.

9. Concerning the colon:

(a) It is retroperitoneal throughout its course.
(b) It is supplied by the superior mesenteric artery only as far as the hepatic flexure.
(c) It is surrounded by a continuous layer of longitudinal and circular muscle.
(d) The sigmoid colon is closely related to the left ureter.
(e) Appendices epiploicae are more frequent in the sigmoid and descending colons compared with the ascending colon.

10. Regarding the liver:

(a) It is completely covered by peritoneum except over its anterior surface.
(b) The hepatic artery, hepatic vein, and bile duct enter and leave the liver at the porta hepatis.
(c) The foetal ductus venosus is represented by the ligamentum teres in the adult.
(d) Venous blood from the liver enters the inferior vena cava via the portal vein.
(e) It receives its arterial supply from a branch of the coeliac trunk.

11. Concerning the gall bladder and biliary system:

(a) The bile duct is formed by the union of the cystic duct with the common hepatic duct.
(b) The bile duct unites with the pancreatic duct to drain into the third part of the duodenum.
(c) The gall bladder is supplied by a branch of the left hepatic artery.
(d) The fundus of the gall bladder lies at the level of the tip of the 9th costal cartilage.
(e) The gall bladder is lined by transitional epithelium.

12. Regarding the kidneys and suprarenal glands:

(a) The right kidney is lower than the left kidney.
(b) The ureter lies anterior to the renal artery and vein at the renal pelvis.
(c) The kidneys are both retroperitoneal.
(d) The suprarenal gland receives its blood from the suprarenal artery only.
(e) The suprarenal gland is innervated from the abdominal sympathetic trunk.

13. Regarding the abdominal blood vessels:

(a) The abdominal aorta ends at the level of L4 vertebra by dividing into the common iliac arteries.
(b) The superior mesenteric artery arises from the aorta at the level of L2 vertebra.
(c) The inferior mesenteric artery supplies the derivatives of the hindgut.
(d) The inferior vena cava drains the two gonadal veins directly.
(e) There are numerous anastomoses of blood vessels supplying the appendix.

14. Concerning the nerves of the abdomen:

(a) The lumbar plexus is formed by the anterior rami of L1–L4 spinal nerves.
(b) The femoral nerve and the obturator nerve lie medial to psoas major.
(c) The iliohypogastric and ilioinguinal nerves arise from L1 spinal nerve.
(d) The genitofemoral nerve is involved in the cremasteric reflex.
(e) The obturator nerve is sensory to the medial aspect of the thigh.

15. Regarding the bones of the upper limb:

(a) The scapula helps to increase the range of movement of the shoulder joint.
(b) The triceps muscle is attached to the coracoid process of the scapula and the humerus.
(c) Fracture of the surgical neck of the humerus may result in injury to the axillary nerve.
(d) The glenoid cavity is surrounded by a rim of cartilage, the glenoid labrum, which is deficient inferiorly.
(e) The radial nerve runs in the spiral groove of the radius.

16. Concerning the joints of the upper limb:

(a) In the adult they are all synovial joints (except the interosseus membrane if included as a joint).
(b) The shoulder joint is completely surrounded by the rotator cuff of muscles.
(c) The shoulder joint relies greatly on the glenohumeral ligaments for stability.
(d) Abduction of the shoulder joint is performed by the deltoid and infraspinatus muscles.
(e) The sternoclavicular joint has an intra-articular disc.

17. Regarding the vessels of the upper limb:

(a) The axillary artery becomes the brachial artery at the inferior border of teres minor.
(b) The brachial artery is superficial throughout most of its course.
(c) The radial artery may be palpated in the anatomical snuffbox.
(d) The ulnar artery runs lateral to the ulnar nerve in the wrist region.
(e) The common interosseous artery arises from the ulnar artery just before it enters the hand.

18. Concerning the nerves of the upper limb:

(a) Damage to the radial nerve results in severe sensory loss in the hands.
(b) The radial nerve supplies the extensor compartment of the arm.
(c) The posterior cutaneous nerve of the forearm is given off by the radial nerve just below the elbow joint.
(d) The axillary nerve arises from the posterior cord of the brachial plexus.
(e) The musculocutaneous nerve is motor to the flexor muscles of the arm.

19. Regarding the nerves of the upper limb:

(a) The median nerve is easily damaged as it crosses the wrist.
(b) The median nerve supplies all the muscles of the thenar eminence.
(c) The median and ulnar nerves give off no branches in the axilla.
(d) The median and radial nerves supply flexor digitorum profundus muscles.
(e) The ulnar nerve is motor to all the interossei muscles of the hand.

183

20. Concerning the muscles of the upper limb:

(a) The supinator muscle forms the floor of the cubital fossa.
(b) The median nerve and ulnar artery pass into the forearm between the origins of flexor digitorum superficialis.
(c) The median nerve passes deep to the two heads of pronator teres as it leaves the cubital fossa.
(d) The ulnar nerve enters the forearm superficial to the two heads of flexor carpi ulnaris.
(e) The deltoid muscle is supplied by the axillary nerve.

21. Concerning bones of the lower limb:

(a) At puberty the three bones of the hip are separated by a Y-shaped cartilage in the acetabulum.
(b) The median sacral crest represents the fused spinal processes of the sacral vertebrae.
(c) The greater sciatic notch is only formed by the posterior margin of the ischium.
(d) The greater trochanter of the femur gives attachment to the piriformis muscle.
(e) The obturator foramen transmits the obturator artery and nerve.

22. Regarding joints of the lower limb:

(a) The close fit of the femoral head in the acetabulum contributes greatly to stability of the hip joint.
(b) Abduction of the hip is performed by gluteus medius and minimus.
(c) Only flexion and extension movements are possible at the knee joint.
(d) The cavity of the knee joint communicates with the suprapatellar bursa.
(e) Extension of the knee joint is performed by the quadriceps femoris muscle.

23. Regarding the femoral triangle:

(a) The femoral vein, artery, and nerve lie in the femoral sheath.
(b) The femoral nerve lies most medially in the femoral triangle.
(c) The lateral border of the femoral triangle is formed by the lateral border of sartorius muscle.
(d) The femoral canal lies medial to the femoral vein.
(e) At the apex of the femoral triangle the femoral vessels pass into the adductor canal.

24. Regarding vessels of the lower limb:

(a) The femoral artery is a direct continuation of the internal iliac artery as it passes below the inguinal ligament.
(b) The profunda femoris artery supplies the muscles of the medial and posterior compartments of the thigh.
(c) The popliteal artery has no branches in the popliteal fossa.
(d) The dorsalis pedis artery is a continuation of the anterior tibial artery in the foot.
(e) The posterior tibial artery may be palpated behind the lateral malleolus.

25. Concerning nerves of the lower limb:

(a) The obturator nerve supplies the muscles of the adductor compartment of the thigh.
(b) The sciatic nerve leaves the pelvis via the greater sciatic foramen.
(c) The femoral nerve is formed from the ventral rami of the L3–L5 spinal nerves.
(d) The superior gluteal nerve supplies the gluteus maximus muscle.
(e) The sciatic nerve may be damaged by posterior dislocation of the hip joint.

26. Concerning nerves of the lower limb:

(a) The tibial nerve ends by dividing into medial and lateral plantar nerves.
(b) Trauma to the common peroneal nerve results in footdrop.
(c) The saphenous nerve passes behind the medial malleolus to supply the medial side of the foot.
(d) The sciatic nerve enters the thigh at the upper border of the piriformis muscle.
(e) The femoral nerve supplies the anterior compartment of the thigh.

27. Concerning the rectum:

(a) It commences where the sigmoid mesocolon ends.
(b) Venous drainage is into the systemic and portal venous systems.
(c) It usually has three permanent transverse folds.
(d) The rectovesical pouch in the female separates the rectum from the bladder.
(e) The mucosa is non-keratinizing, stratified squamous epithelium.

28. Regarding pelvic structures:

(a) The bladder is covered by peritoneum on its superior surface.
(b) The broad ligament of the uterus contains the fallopian tubes and ovarian vessels.
(c) The ovary lies on the posterior surface of the broad ligament.
(d) The transverse cervical ligaments play a part in the stabilization of the uterus.
(e) The posterior fornix of the vagina is deeper than the anterior fornix.

29. Concerning vessels of the pelvis:

(a) The ovarian artery arises from the internal iliac artery.
(b) The internal pudendal artery leaves the pelvis through the lesser sciatic foramen.
(c) The obturator artery is crossed laterally by the ureter.
(d) The uterine artery may anastomose with the ovarian artery and the vaginal artery.
(e) The uterine artery is closely related to the ureter just before it reaches the uterus.

30. Regarding the perineum:

(a) The external anal sphincter is formed by two muscle layers.
(b) Voluntary contraction of the external anal sphincter may delay defaecation.
(c) The entire anal canal is supplied by the autonomic nervous system.
(d) The dorsal artery of the penis assists in supplying the skin and superficial tissues of the penis.
(e) The pudendal nerve supplies the lower part of the vagina.

31. Concerning the face and scalp:

(a) The buccal branch of the facial nerve is sensory to the buccal mucosa.
(b) The muscles of facial expression lie below the deep fascia of the face.
(c) The trigeminal nerve is sensory to the entire scalp region.
(d) The facial vein is formed by the union of the supraorbital and supratrochlear veins.
(e) The arterial supply to the face and scalp is from branches of the external carotid artery only.

32. Regarding the salivary glands:

(a) The external carotid artery and the retromandibular vein lie in the substance of the parotid gland.
(b) The parotid duct opens in the oral cavity opposite the second premolar tooth.
(c) The facial nerve gives off its five terminal branches before it enters the parotid gland.
(d) The superficial and deep parts of the submandibular gland are continuous around the mylohyoid muscle.
(e) Paraesthesia to the tongue may result following surgery to the sublingual glands.

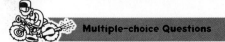

33. Concerning the larynx:

(a) The sensory nerve supply to the mucosa of the larynx above the level of the vocal folds is from the recurrent laryngeal nerve.
(b) The cricothyroid muscle is supplied by the internal laryngeal nerve.
(c) The epiglottis is composed of elastic cartilage.
(d) The vocal membrane is the thickened upper edge of the cricothyroid ligament.
(e) The posterior cricoarytenoid muscle abducts the vocal folds.

34. Concerning the cranial cavity:

(a) The tentorium cerebelli forms a roof over the posterior cranial fossa.
(b) The sigmoid venous sinus becomes the internal jugular vein at the jugular foramen.
(c) Infection in the infraorbital region may spread to the cavernous sinus.
(d) The circulus arteriosus connects the internal and external carotid arteries.
(e) The internal carotid artery and the trochlear nerve run through the cavernous sinus.

35. Concerning the orbit:

(a) The central artery of the retina is an end artery.
(b) The superior rectus muscle is supplied by the trochlear nerve.
(c) Levator palpebrae superioris has a somatic and autonomic nerve supply.
(d) Inferior oblique moves the cornea inferiorly and laterally.
(e) The inferior orbital fissure communicates with the pterygopalatine fossa.

36. Concerning the oral cavity:

(a) Sensation to the anterior two-thirds of the tongue is supplied by the lingual nerve.
(b) The vallate papillae lie just posterior to the sulcus terminalis.
(c) The hard palate is formed by the horizontal process of the palatine bones alone.
(d) The extrinsic muscles of the tongue are supplied by the lingual nerve.
(e) The foramen caecum on the tongue is the embryological remnant marking the site of the upper end of the thyroglossal duct.

37. In the neck region:

(a) The external jugular vein is formed by the union of the posterior auricular vein and posterior division of the retromandibular vein.
(b) The accessory nerve supplies the trapezius muscle.
(c) The digastric muscle is supplied by the facial nerve only.
(d) The thyrohyoid muscle is supplied by the recurrent laryngeal nerve.
(e) The superior thyroid artery arises from the posterior aspect of the external carotid artery.

38. Concerning the neck:

(a) The investing layer of deep fascia forms the sphenomandibular ligament.
(b) The cervical plexus is formed by the anterior rami of C1–C4 spinal nerves.
(c) The pretracheal fascia blends with the fibrous pericardium inferiorly.
(d) The internal carotid artery has only two branches in the neck.
(e) The deep cervical lymph nodes lie along the posterior border of sternomastoid.

39. Concerning the bones of the skull and face:

(a) The lateral pterygoid muscle is attached to the coronoid process of the mandible.

(b) The maxilla takes part in the formation of the hard palate.

(c) The lingual nerve may be damaged during the removal of a mandibular third molar tooth.

(d) The temporal bone transmits the VII and VIII cranial nerves.

(e) The nasal septum is completely cartilaginous.

40. Regarding the cranial nerves:

(a) The optic nerve is accompanied by the ophthalmic artery through the optic canal.

(b) The cranial part of the accessory nerve is sensory to the mucosa of the pharynx.

(c) The trigeminal nerve is motor to the muscles of mastication.

(d) The oculomotor nerve transmits parasympathetic fibres to the lacrimal gland.

(e) The facial nerve transmits taste fibres from the posterior third of the tongue.

1. Draw a diagram to illustrate the components and branches of the cervical plexus.

2. Describe the innervation of the mucosa of the tongue.

3. List the lymphatic drainage of the pelvis.

4. Illustrate the components of the rectus sheath.

5. Briefly describe the arterial blood supply of the heart.

6. List the muscles, vessels, and nerves of a typical intercostal space.

7. Describe the origin, course, and distribution of the obturator nerve.

8. Describe the first cervical vertebra.

9. Write short notes on the biceps brachii muscle.

10. Describe the borders and contents of the femoral triangle.

11. Briefly describe the uterine tubes.

12. Describe the flexor retinaculum of the wrist, including its bony attachments, and the contents of the carpal tunnel.

Essay Questions

1. Describe the origin, course, and distribution of the median nerve.

2. Describe the course and distribution of the thoracic aorta.

3. Discuss the muscular attachments of the diaphragm and the structures passing through it.

4. Describe the anatomy of the inguinal canal and its contents.

5. Discuss the course and distribution of the superior mesenteric artery.

6. Summarize the autonomic nerve supply of the pelvis.

7. Describe the course and distribution of the sciatic nerve.

8. Describe the fascial layers of the neck.

9. Discuss the muscles of mastication, including their nerve supply.

10. Describe the origin and distribution of the facial nerve.

MCQ Answers

1. (a) T, (b) F, (c) T, (d) F, (e) F
2. (a) F, (b) T, (c) T, (d) T, (e) T
3. (a) F, (b) F, (c) T, (d) T, (e) F
4. (a) F, (b) T, (c) T, (d) F, (e) F
5. (a) T, (b) F, (c) F, (d) F, (e) F
6. (a) T, (b) T, (c) F, (d) F, (e) F
7. (a) T, (b) F, (c) F, (d) F, (e) T
8. (a) T, (b) T, (c) F, (d) T, (e) F
9. (a) F, (b) F, (c) F, (d) T, (e) T
10. (a) F, (b) F, (c) F, (d) F, (e) T
11. (a) T, (b) F, (c) F, (d) T, (e) F
12. (a) T, (b) F, (c) T, (d) F, (e) F
13. (a) T, (b) F, (c) T, (d) F, (e) F
14. (a) T, (b) F, (c) T, (d) T, (e) T
15. (a) T, (b) F, (c) T, (d) F, (e) F
16. (a) T, (b) F, (c) F, (d) F, (e) T
17. (a) F, (b) T, (c) T, (d) T, (e) F
18. (a) F, (b) T, (c) F, (d) T, (e) T
19. (a) T, (b) T, (c) T, (d) F, (e) T
20. (a) T, (b) T, (c) T, (d) F, (e) T

21. (a) T, (b) T, (c) F, (d) T, (e) T
22. (a) T, (b) T, (c) F, (d) T, (e) T
23. (a) F, (b) F, (c) F, (d) T, (e) T
24. (a) F, (b) T, (c) F, (d) T, (e) F
25. (a) T, (b) T, (c) F, (d) F, (e) T
26. (a) T, (b) T, (c) F, (d) F, (e) T
27. (a) T, (b) T, (c) T, (d) F, (e) F
28. (a) T, (b) T, (c) T, (d) T, (e) T
29. (a) F, (b) F, (c) F, (d) T, (e) T
30. (a) F, (b) T, (c) F, (d) T, (e) T
31. (a) F, (b) F, (c) F, (d) T, (e) F
32. (a) T, (b) F, (c) F, (d) T, (e) T
33. (a) F, (b) F, (c) T, (d) T, (e) T
34. (a) T, (b) T, (c) T, (d) F, (e) F
35. (a) T, (b) F, (c) T, (d) F, (e) T
36. (a) T, (b) F, (c) F, (d) F, (e) T
37. (a) T, (b) T, (c) F, (d) F, (e) F
38. (a) F, (b) T, (c) T, (d) F, (e) F
39. (a) F, (b) T, (c) T, (d) T, (e) F
40. (a) T, (b) F, (c) T, (d) F, (e) F

SAQ Answers

1. See Fig. 7.51.

2. The mucosa of the tongue has sensory fibres that supply the special sense of taste, as well as sensations of pain, temperature, and touch. The salivary glands of the tongue are also supplied by parasympathetic secretomotor fibres.

   For the anterior two-thirds of the tongue, fibres of common sensation are carried to the trigeminal ganglion via the lingual nerve. Taste fibres travel in the lingual nerve and then in the chorda tympani and facial nerve, to the geniculate ganglion of the facial nerve. Parasympathetic secretomotor fibres from the superior salivary nucleus of the facial nerve pass via the chorda tympani and lingual nerve to synapse in the submandibular ganglion. Postganglionic fibres join the lingual nerve again and supply the glands of the anterior two-thirds of the tongue.

   All sensation to the posterior third of the tongue and to the vallate papillae is supplied by the lingual branch of the glossopharyngeal nerve.

3. See Fig 5.21.

4. See Fig. 4.5.

5. The heart is supplied by the right and left coronary arteries. Because the blood vessels of the heart are compressed during systole, blood flows in these vessels only in diastole.

   The right coronary artery arises from the right anterior aortic sinus. It runs down in the coronary sulcus, which leads to the inferior margin of the heart. Here it anastomoses with the circumflex branch of the left coronary artery before running forward to the apex as the posterior interventricular artery. It gives off the marginal artery, as well as branches to the right atrium and right ventricle.

   The left coronary artery arises from the left anterior aortic sinus and passes forwards between the pulmonary trunk and the left auricle and divides into the circumflex artery and the anterior interventricular artery. The circumflex artery runs in the atrioventricular sulcus posteriorly to anastomose with the right coronary artery.

It gives off branches to the atria and the left ventricle. The anterior interventricular artery descends in the anterior interventricular sulcus towards the apex of the heart. It gives branches to the right and left ventricles and the interventricular septum.

   The distribution described is the one most commonly found; however, variation is not uncommon.

6. The muscles of an intercostal space are the external intercostal, internal intercostal, and innermost intercostal. They are all supplied by the intercostal nerves. Their functions are to elevate and depress the ribs during external respiration.

   The vessels of an intercostal space are the posterior and anterior intercostal arteries. Posterior intercostals, spaces 1–2, originate from the superior intercostal artery and a branch of the costocervical trunk of the subclavian artery; posterior intercostals, lower 9 spaces, originate from the thoracic aorta. Anterior intercostals, spaces 1–9, originate from the internal thoracic artery; anterior intercostals, spaces 7–9, originate from the musculophrenic artery, a branch of the internal thoracic artery. Each artery supplies the skin, muscles, and parietal pleura.

   The intercostal nerves are the anterior rami of the upper thoracic spinal nerves. The first six nerves are distributed within their intercostal spaces. The other nerves pass to the anterior abdominal wall. They supply the skin, parietal pleura, and intercostal muscles.

   The nerves and vessels are protected by the subcostal groove of the ribs. This neuromuscular bundle runs between the second (internal intercostal) and third (transversus thoracic) muscle layers.

7. The obturator nerve (L2–L4) arises from the lumbar plexus. It divides into anterior and posterior branches and runs with the obturator artery through the obturator canal to supply the obturator externus muscle and the hip joint.

   The anterior branch passes anterior to adductor brevis and supplies this muscle, together with adductor longus and gracilis. The nerve continues to supply the skin of the medial aspect of the thigh.

   The posterior branch passes behind the adductor

brevis to supply adductor magnus and the knee joint.

In the pelvis the nerve is closely associated with the ovary, and ovarian pathology may cause referred pain to the medial aspect of the thigh.

8. The first cervical vertebra or atlas is composed of two lateral masses joined by anterior and posterior arches. The posterior arch has a small posterior tubercle, but there is no body or spinous process.

The atlas has facets on the superior and inferior surfaces of the lateral masses, which articulate with the occipital condyles superiorly and with the superior articular facets of the axis inferiorly. The anterior arch has a small facet for articulation with the dens or odontoid process of the axis. These are all synovial joints.

On the medial aspect of each lateral mass is a small tubercle for attachment of the transverse ligament of the atlas.

The atlanto-occipital joints allow flexion and extension movements of the head, whereas the head and the atlas rotate around the atlantoaxial joints.

9. This is a muscle of the anterior or flexor compartment of the arm. It has two heads. The long head originates from the supraglenoid tubercle of the scapula within the capsule of the shoulder joint. It emerges from the capsule between the greater and lesser tubercles of the humerus and passes down in the intertubercular sulcus. The short head arises from the coracoid process of the scapula.

The two muscle bellies fuse in the lower part of the arm and give rise to a tendon that is attached to the tuberosity of the radius. As the tendon crosses the elbow joint, the bicipital aponeurosis crosses medially over the brachial artery to fuse with the deep fascia of the arm.

The muscle is supplied by the musculocutaneous nerve. It is a powerful flexor and supinator of the elbow joint and a flexor of the shoulder joint.

10. The femoral triangle is formed by the inguinal ligament, the sartorius muscle, and the adductor longus muscle. The floor is formed by the iliopsoas and pectineus muscles, and the roof by the fascia lata and cribriform fascia.

From lateral to medial, the triangle contains the femoral nerve, femoral artery, femoral vein, and the femoral canal. Medial to the femoral canal is the lacunar ligament. The femoral artery and vein and the femoral canal are enclosed within a thickened fascial sheath, the femoral sheath. The femoral artery gives off its profunda femoris branch at the apex of the triangle. The femoral triangle also contains deep lymph nodes associated with the femoral vein. At the apex of the triangle the femoral vessels pass into the adductor canal.

11. The uterine tubes arise from the junction of the body and fundus of the uterus. They lie in the superior border of the broad ligament. The isthmus is the most medial and narrow part of the tube and communicates with the uterine cavity. More laterally the tube expands to form the ampulla—this passes posteriorly to end close to the superior aspect of the ovary as the infundibulum. The latter has several processes called fimbriae. one of which is attached to the ovary.

The ovary releases an ovum into the peritoneal cavity. This passes into the infundibulum and then into the uterine cavity. Fertilization usually occurs in the uterine tubes.

The blood supply of the tubes is from the ovarian artery and the uterine artery.

12. The flexor retinaculum is a strong band of fibrous tissue that serves to bind the long flexor tendons of the forearm, preventing them from bowing when the wrist is flexed. It is attached to the pisiform bone and the hook of hamate medially and the tubercle of the scaphoid and trapezium laterally. The osseofibrous tunnel (the carpal tunnel) thus formed allows passage of the long flexor tendons of the wrist in their synovial sheaths and the median nerve.

The short muscles of the hand that make up the thenar and hypothenar eminences arise from the flexor retinaculum.

Compression of the median nerve in the carpal tunnel is a common clinical condition. It may be relieved by cutting the flexor retinaculum to relieve the tension on the nerve.

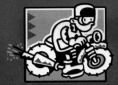

Index

Specific arteries, muscles, nerves, and veins are listed under their individual full names, not grouped under general entries.